THE CORTISOL CONSPIRACY

You're Not Stressed—You're Addicted

How Cortisol Became the Brain's Legal Drug—Fueling Burnout, Fatigue, and Anxiety, and How to Break the Cycle for Good

Copyright © 2025 by Bendjedith Momo, PhD.
All rights reserved. No part of this book may be reproduced, stored in a retrieval system, or transmitted in any form or by any means—electronic, mechanical, photocopying, recording, or otherwise—without the prior written permission of the publisher, except in the case of brief quotations used in critical articles or reviews.

First edition published by Bendjedith Momo Dongmo, PhD.
www.mbcglobalmedia.com
bendjedithpublishing@yahoo.com

ISBN (Paperback): 979-8-9990659-0-2

ISBN (Hardback): 979-8-9990659-1-9

ISBN (Ebook): 979-8-9990659-2-6

Printed in the United States of America
10 9 8 7 6 5 4 3 2 1

Disclaimer:
The author and publisher are not engaged in rendering medical, psychological, or other professional services. The content presented in this book is intended for informational and educational purposes only and should not be considered a substitute for professional medical advice, diagnosis, or treatment. Readers are advised to consult a licensed healthcare provider for individual guidance.

CONTENTS

Introduction: The Lie You've Been Living..................................5
  Why Exhaustion Feels Normal—and Why You Should Be Scared

PART I: THE NEUROCHEMICAL PRISON...............9

Chapter 1: The Hidden High 10
  The Drug You Never Chose—How Your Own Body Hooked You on the World's Most Dangerous High

Chapter 2: The Burnout Business Model 39
  Stress for Sale—How Corporations Turned Your Burnout Into Billions

Chapter 3: The Dopamine-Cortisol Trap 71
  Why Rest Feels Like Withdrawal— The Hidden Neuroscience of Why You Can't Relax

PART II: THE HIDDEN COSTS OF ADDICTION 98

Chapter 4: Your Stolen Energy..99
  Stolen Life—The Silent Energy Drains Killing Your Vitality

Chapter 5: The Relationship Killer...132
  The Love You Lost to Cortisol—How Stress Destroys Relationships Before It Destroys You

Chapter 6: The Cortisol Debt..176
  The Debt You Didn't Know You Owed—Every Stressful Day Lives in Your Body, and It's Time to Pay the Bill

PART III: THE ESCAPE PLAN 218

Chapter 7: Rebuilding Without Stress 219
Break the Cycle—The Revolutionary Blueprint to Rewire Your Brain and Reclaim Your Life

Chapter 8: Cortisol Fasting 248
Fasting from Stress—How I Survived Collapse and Turned My Nervous System Into an Ally

Chapter 9: The Cortisol Mastery Blueprint 279
Mastery Over Cortisol—How to Turn Your Greatest Enemy Into Your Superpower

Master Chapter: The Future of Cortisol Control 314
The Global Awakening—Why Fortune 500 Companies Are Quietly Learning This and Why You Can't Afford to Ignore It

Conclusion: Your Choice 343
Choose Your Ending—You Can Keep Surviving, or You Can Finally Start Living

INTRODUCTION:
THE LIE YOU'VE BEEN LIVING

*Why Exhaustion Feels Normal—and Why
You Should Be Scared*

You're exhausted, but you can't sleep.

You've been staring at the ceiling for hours, your mind racing through tomorrow's to-do list, replaying today's meetings, and cycling through the endless responsibilities waiting for you when the sun rises. Your body is tired—bone tired—but your brain won't shut off.

This isn't just a bad night. This is your life now.

Maybe you've started to wonder if something is wrong with you. Why can't you handle what everyone else seems to manage effortlessly? Why do you feel drained even after a full night's sleep? Why does your success feel increasingly hollow, your relationships increasingly distant, and your life increasingly like something you're watching rather than living?

It's not you. It's the trap you never saw coming.

You're caught in a biochemical addiction that society has convinced you is normal. You're trapped in a cycle so pervasive that we've built our entire economy around it. You're hooked on a drug that's destroying you—and we call it "ambition," "dedication," or "work ethic."

That drug is stress. And it's killing you, one cortisol spike at a time.

For years, I thought my exhaustion was a personal failure. I pushed harder, stayed later at the office, checked emails at midnight, and wore my exhaustion like a badge of honor. I believed the lie that success required sacrifice, that stress was the price of achievement, and that burnout was just a phase I needed to push through.

I was wrong.

What I discovered instead was something the most successful people in the world already know: **Stress isn't fuel for success—it's what's holding you back from your highest potential.**

The truth is that your brain on chronic stress is operating at a fraction of its capability. Your creativity is stunted, your decision-making is compromised, and your energy is constantly being drained by a system that was never designed to run on high alert 24/7.

Science now proves what your body has been trying to tell you: You weren't built to live this way.

But here's what no one tells you: There's a way out.

Not just a temporary escape—a complete reset of your relationship with stress. A way to perform at levels you've never experienced before, without the constant drain of cortisol and adrenaline. A system where success doesn't require suffering, where achievement doesn't demand exhaustion, and where your best work comes from a place of calm power, not desperate pushing.

This isn't about meditation apps or weekend retreats that temporarily lower your stress levels before you dive back into the same broken system. This is about breaking free from the addiction itself.

In this book, I'll show you how to:

- Recognize the hidden signs that stress is controlling you—even when you think you're in control
- Break the biochemical addiction that makes your brain crave chaos and urgency
- Reset your nervous system to function at its highest level—without the cortisol spikes
- Build systems that make stress irrelevant, not just manageable
- Create success that energizes you rather than depletes you

What you're about to read isn't just another self-help book about burnout. It's a complete rewiring of how you understand performance, productivity, and potential. It's the science of how your body is meant to function—and how to get back to that optimal state.

The world doesn't need another burnt-out high achiever. It needs what you're capable of when you're operating at your full capacity—clear, focused, and free from the addiction that's been holding you back.

The journey we're about to take goes against everything modern society has taught you about success. It challenges the fundamental belief that stress is necessary for achievement. And it reveals a truth that will change everything: **Your highest performance comes when stress is no longer running the show.**

Turn the page, and let's break free.

It's time to discover who you are without stress as your fuel.

PART I:

THE NEUROCHEMICAL PRISON

CHAPTER 1:
THE HIDDEN HIGH

The Drug You Never Chose—How Your Own Body Hooked You on the World's Most Dangerous High

The day Rachel Summers finally broke wasn't the day she collapsed.

It was a Tuesday afternoon when everything was going right.

Her presentation had impressed the executive team. Her inbox was—miraculously—under control. Her son's teacher had called with glowing feedback. By every measure, this should have been a good day.

Yet as she sat in her sleek corner office at Vertex Media, a strange hollowness spread through her chest. Her hands trembled slightly. Her breathing felt shallow. A voice in her head whispered that something was terribly wrong, though she couldn't name what.

When the panic attack hit, it wasn't triggered by crisis—but by its absence.

Rachel didn't need a therapist to tell her this wasn't normal. What she didn't understand was the truth that would eventually save her life: she wasn't suffering from stress.

She was suffering from its withdrawal.

Like millions of high-achievers, Rachel wasn't just experiencing burnout. She was addicted to stress—her brain chemically dependent on the very thing destroying her. And like any addiction, the damage wasn't in the high, but in what it was quietly stealing from her.
Her health. Her relationships. Her ability to feel joy without urgency as its trigger.

This isn't just Rachel's story. It's an epidemic hiding in plain sight—disguised as ambition, celebrated as work ethic, and destroying lives one promotion at a time.

The most dangerous addiction in modern life isn't to substances. It's to stress itself.

And the conspiracy keeping us hooked runs deeper than you think.

How Stress Became Her Fuel

Rachel hadn't always lived this way.

Once, work had boundaries—concrete edges that separated professional from personal. But as she climbed through Vertex's ranks, from junior copywriter to team lead to executive, patterns emerged that couldn't be ignored. Success wasn't measured by innovation or insight. Instead, it lived in the shadows of midnight emails and canceled vacations. The people who advanced weren't the visionaries—they were the ones who never stopped moving.

Emails at midnight? Dedication personified. Vacations abandoned? Commitment incarnate. Perpetual busyness? The mark of excellence.

The unspoken rule pulsed through the company culture: **exhaustion equals success**. And so, Rachel adapted with terrifying efficiency.

Her desk light remained on long after others had left, casting a lonely glow across abandoned workstations. Her phone never silenced, even during her son's bedtime stories. She thrived in the chaos because in her world, stillness meant irrelevance. Calm meant falling behind while others raced ahead.

She told herself she controlled this rhythm. The truth lurked beneath her self-deception: stress had its fingers wrapped around every aspect of her existence, squeezing tighter with each passing day.

The First Signs of Withdrawal

Waves crashed against pristine sand, their rhythm steady and soothing—everything Rachel's life was not. This was supposed to be freedom: a beachfront villa, no laptop, no calls—just rest.
Instead, panic clawed at her chest.

Her fingers twitched toward her phone every few minutes, phantom vibrations haunting her even when it remained silent. Guilt crushed her for each hour spent unproductively. Her body, accustomed to constant adrenaline, rebelled against relaxation—muscles tight, mind racing, heart pounding with invisible urgency.

That's when realization struck like lightning on a clear day. This wasn't just a habit she'd developed.

This was addiction.

Her brain had rewired itself to survive on urgency, to need adrenaline just to function. Now, deprived of her chemical cocktail, she spiraled into the disorienting abyss of withdrawal.

The Dopamine-Cortisol Loop: Why You Can't Stop

Most people conceptualize addiction through substances—alcohol, opioids, and nicotine. But Rachel's addiction operated on a more fundamental level, a biochemical dependency as real as any drug.

Dopamine — The Chase Chemical.

The office buzzed with its invisible presence, fueling Rachel's exhilaration of almost crossing the finish line. It kept Rachel chasing the next task, the next goal, the next deadline—a hamster wheel that never stopped turning. The irony twisted like a knife: finishing things felt inexplicably anticlimactic because the thrill lived in the pursuit, not the completion.

Cortisol — The Stress Hormone.

It flooded her system daily, maintaining her perpetual high-alert status. Fight-or-flight responses are triggered over minor setbacks, transforming everyday challenges into emergencies. Over time, her brain grew desensitized, requiring increasingly stressful situations to feel engaged. Yesterday's crisis became today's normal, tomorrow's insufficient stimulus.

This is why stress feels productive.

Rachel didn't consciously want to drown in overwhelm. Her brain had simply learned to need it, the way lungs need oxygen—an essential element for survival in her distorted reality.

The Workplace That Kept Her Hooked

Vertex Media's sleek glass headquarters didn't just house stress—its very architecture and culture were designed to maintain addiction.

Emails multiplied like cells dividing. Last-minute "urgent" requests dropped from senior management without warning. The culture celebrated those who sacrificed everything while whispering about those who dared to maintain boundaries.

This wasn't a flaw in the system. It was the system's foundation.

A stressed workforce is an obedient workforce.

Exhausted employees lack the energy to push back against unreasonable demands. Overwhelmed workers don't negotiate for better conditions. People addicted to stress continue feeding the machine that slowly consumes them, mistaking exploitation for opportunity.

Rachel wasn't just an addict. She was the perfect corporate asset—until the inevitable crash began.

The First Crack in the System

The breakdown didn't announce itself with dramatic flair.

Instead, it whispered through small fractures in her carefully constructed facade.

Her best friend's birthday passed without acknowledgment, a date once sacred now buried beneath project deadlines. Her son's school play—the one where he had practiced his three lines for weeks—proceeded without her in the audience, her empty seat a void he had already learned to expect. Sharp words escaped her lips toward loved ones, frustration leaking from overfilled emotional reserves.

"I've got this," she repeated like a mantra. "Stress is fuel, not fire."

But one night, alone in her apartment, the blue light of her laptop illuminating her exhausted face as she stared at an inbox that multiplied faster than she could empty it, a question surfaced from somewhere deep within:

What if this isn't making me stronger? What if this is breaking me?

For the first time in years, fear gripped her—not the productive kind that drove her forward, but the paralyzing kind that forced her to see the truth.

The Stress Tolerance Effect

At first, Rachel needed a little pressure to maintain peak performance.

A tight deadline sparked creativity, a fast-paced project brought out her best strategic thinking, and a bit of chaos made her feel alive and necessary.

But soon, insidiously, the baseline shifted.

Standard workloads evoked boredom rather than focus. Normal stress levels barely registered in her awareness. She needed—craved—more urgency, crises, and fires to extinguish just to feel like herself.

This is the truth about stress addiction that employee wellness programs never address: The more stress you experience, the more stress you need to function.

Until suddenly—inevitably— **Calm doesn't feel like calm anymore. It feels like withdrawal.**

Parenting on Empty

Five-year-old Ethan's world revolved around dinosaurs, superheroes, and the increasingly rare moments when his mother was truly present. Rachel wasn't just failing herself. The collateral damage extended to the small human who needed her most.

He had stopped asking whether she'd make his soccer games, his hope extinguished by too many broken promises. His artwork remained unshared, colorful masterpieces hidden away to protect them from her distracted glances. At five years old, he had internalized a devastating lesson: Mommy's attention was a limited resource for which he had to compete—and usually lose.

The night he finally stopped waiting for her to tuck him in and continued his bedtime routine without her, something inside Rachel shattered.

What if I don't just lose my health? What if I lose him, too?

That night, emails remained unchecked. Her laptop stayed closed. For the first time in years, she sat with the uncomfortable stillness of her own thoughts and asked the question that terrified her most:

If stress isn't my fuel... what is?

The Cost of Control

Rachel's addiction to stress had metastasized beyond her job at Vertex. It had become her entire operating system, her very way of being in the world.

Her body had forgotten how to function without crisis—the quiet moments felt wrong, dangerous even. High stakes made colors appear brighter, sounds sharper. Urgency transformed mundane tasks into missions of critical importance. Chaos whispered seductive reassurances that she mattered, that she was essential, irreplaceable.

But the cracks in her foundation grew wider by the day.

Exhaustion clung to her like a second skin, no amount of sleep sufficient to wash it away. Her time with Ethan felt hollow, her physical presence undermined by her mental absence. Even when she managed to step away from work, her nervous system remained charged, hypervigilant, waiting for the next emergency.

The worst revelation? **She had no roadmap for escape.**

The Day Her Body Said 'Enough'

It wasn't the dramatic collapse she might have expected—no ambulance lights, no emergency room, no concerned colleagues gathering around a fallen figure.

Instead, her body staged a quiet rebellion one Tuesday morning.

Sunlight filtered through half-drawn blinds as Rachel blinked awake, immediately aware that something had changed. A strange heaviness pinned her to the mattress, as though gravity had doubled overnight.

Her limbs ignored commands to move, leaden and disconnected. Fog filled her skull where sharp clarity usually resided. Her heart raced erratically, though she hadn't moved an inch.

Get up. Just get up.

The internal command that had always worked now echoed uselessly in her mind.

For years, warning signs had flashed before her—migraines that lasted for days, exhaustion that sleep couldn't touch, irritability that had no specific target, gaps in memory that frightened her in quiet moments.

Now, the bill had come due in full.

She had overdrafted her nervous system.

The Biology of Burnout

Dr. Alexander Hughes, a neuropsychologist specializing in high-performance burnout and stress-related disorders, would later explain to Rachel what happened that morning. Her breakdown wasn't a character flaw or mental weakness. It was a biochemical inevitability— as predictable as physics.

Cortisol Debt — When Your Body Stops Lending You Energy
Initially, stress granted her a false sense of power, allowing her to push beyond normal human limitations. Over time, it systematically drained

her real energy reserves, depleting resources faster than they could replenish. When she pushed too far for too long, her body defaulted on the loan and initiated emergency shutdown protocols.

That's what had happened to Rachel, alone in her bedroom with the weight of exhaustion crushing her chest.

She wasn't lazy. She wasn't weak.

She was running on an empty tank, and her body's emergency reserves had long since been depleted. Despite the overwhelming evidence, a thought surfaced from her stress-addicted brain: *Maybe I just need more coffee.*

The Work-Addict's Excuse

Rachel dragged herself from bed, movements sluggish as though moving through water. The kitchen's harsh light assaulted her eyes as she fumbled with the coffee maker, spilling grounds across the counter.

More caffeine. More adrenaline. More urgency. The formula that had always worked before would surely work again.

Except it didn't.

The coffee sat bitter on her tongue, its promised energy nowhere to be found. Her body remained heavy, unresponsive to the chemical that had reliably jump-started her system for years. Her brain refused to engage, and her thoughts were scattered and incomplete.

What's happening to me?

For the first time in her career, the stress response—her faithful companion and secret weapon—failed to activate.

And that terrified her more than any deadline or crisis ever had.

Had she finally broken herself beyond repair? The question echoed in the empty kitchen, unanswered.

The Missed Wake-Up Calls

Warning signs flashed red for years, and each was dismissed with practiced efficiency.

The migraines that left her vomiting in bathroom stalls between meetings weren't "just stress"—they were her nervous system begging for reprieve. The memory lapses that made her panic briefly before blaming busyness weren't insignificant—they were cognitive function deteriorating under chronic strain. The restless nights staring at dark ceilings weren't "just overthinking"—they were her body too charged to power down.

Voices of concern had surrounded her, each one brushed aside.

Her best friend Emily's worried eyes over rarely-touched lunch.

"You're disappearing, Rach. I barely recognize you anymore."

Her boss, Leila's unexpected concern during their quarterly review.

"You're delivering exceptional work, but at what cost? You look like you need a break."

Ethan's innocent question that should have broken her heart.

"Mommy, why are you always tired? Is it because of me?"

She had constructed elaborate defenses:

I can handle it. I just need to push through. It's just a busy quarter.

But what if her greatest strength—pushing through—had become her most destructive weakness?

Parenting on Auto-Pilot

The breakdown revealed itself most painfully in the small moments with Ethan—precious seconds of connection lost forever.

Bedtime stories once savored are now rushed through, her eyes scanning each page for the fastest route to the end. Soccer games are watched through the filter of work emails, and his triumphant waves toward the bleachers are met with delayed, distracted responses.

Conversations half-heard, questions half-answered, presence half-given—a mother physically there but mentally unreachable.

Ethan was only five—his world still small and centered around her—but he had already adapted to her emotional absence.

He had learned to wait until the laptop closed before showing his drawings. He knew certain phone calls meant playtime ended prematurely. He recognized the glazed look in her eyes, which meant she had heard his words but hadn't absorbed their meaning.

She hadn't intended to push him away. She loved him fiercely, completely.

But stress had made her numb to what mattered most.

The worst realization? She hadn't even noticed the distance growing between them—not until he stopped trying to bridge it.

The Silent Goodbye

One Wednesday evening, Rachel pushed open Ethan's bedroom door, guilt-driven determination to be present for bedtime propelling her forward.

The sight before her stopped her cold.

Ethan lay curled on his side, already asleep. His dinosaur book sprawled open beside him, small fingers still curled around its edge. The night light cast soft shadows across his face, and he turned away from the door as though he'd been watching for someone who never came.

She stood frozen in the doorway, the weight of realization crushing her chest.

When was the last time I tucked him in without checking emails halfway through?

He hadn't called for her. He hadn't waited up. The nighttime ritual they once shared had been modified—he had adapted to her absence by learning to fall asleep alone.

He had stopped expecting her to show up.
And in that moment, watching her son's chest rise and fall in the dim light, Rachel felt something fundamental break inside her—something no promotion or bonus could ever repair.

The Cost of Being 'The Best'

Her entire adult identity had been constructed around achievement.

The best at her job—fourteen awards and three promotions in five years proved it. The most reliable in crisis situations—her phone rang first when campaigns faltered. The hardest worker in every room—her car often the last in Vertex's parking garage.

But what had it cost her?

Her body was shutting down, one system at a time. Her friendships had atrophied from neglect. Her son was learning to live without the full presence of his mother. And for what? Another client? Another campaign? Another line on a resume no one would read at her funeral?

For the first time, success felt hollow—a pyrrhic victory in a war she never needed to fight.

The Withdrawal Nobody Talks About

Rachel had misconceptions about burnout—that it would announce itself dramatically, a definitive moment of collapse she couldn't possibly miss.
Reality proved more insidious.

Burnout doesn't arrive like a thunderclap but erodes you like water shaping stone—patient, persistent, nearly invisible until the damage is done. By the time you recognize the symptoms, you're already deep in its grip.

She had spent years borrowing energy from her future self—living on cortisol loans she could never repay. Now her nervous system had declared bankruptcy, shutting down non-essential functions to preserve basic operations.

But the cruelest revelation came next:

Quitting stress felt worse than living in it.

The First Day Without the Rush

After a frank conversation with Dr. Hughes, Rachel committed to breaking her stress addiction.

No email before breakfast. Coffee is limited to one cup, consumed slowly. No reactive work until she'd set intentions for the day.

The plan seemed solid, grounded in neuroscience and recovery principles. But as she sat at her kitchen table that morning, staring at her untouched phone, unexpected discomfort crawled beneath her skin.

Restlessness pulsed through her chest. Her thoughts scattered without the focusing lens of urgency. A physical craving stronger than hunger gnawed at her resolve.

This is ridiculous. I have responsibilities.

Her fingers twitched toward the phone, muscle memory stronger than conscious choice.

Just one email. Just a quick check.

She forced her hand back to her lap, breathing through the discomfort. The silence of her apartment felt oppressive, wrong. Her body physically ached for the chemical rush; she'd denied it.

This wasn't relief. This was **withdrawal**.

Her symptoms paralleled those of a drug addict detoxing—and Dr. Hughes had warned this would be the hardest part. The body fights for homeostasis, even when that balance point is dangerously unhealthy.

Why Quitting Stress Feels Like Losing Yourself

Rachel had built her entire identity around being busy, needed, essential.

The problem solver who never failed. The executive who handled impossible situations with grace. The person colleagues and clients counted on when everything went wrong.

If she stopped? **Who would she be without the pressure that had defined her?**

This is the aspect of burnout recovery that wellness retreats and self-care articles rarely address.

People assume escaping burnout is primarily about rest and recovery. But the deeper challenge is identity reconstruction.

It's about grieving the person stress made you into—the capabilities, the recognition, the worth you believed came from your capacity to endure. It's about learning to exist without the chaos that gave your days structure and meaning. It's about becoming someone new when you've invested years in perfecting who you were—and that transformation is terrifying.

The Unraveling

By noon, Rachel's resolve crumbled beneath the weight of withdrawal.

She grabbed her laptop, justifications flowing freely as she opened her email. "Just checking in," she told herself. "Just being responsible."

The inbox that usually overflowed with emergencies displayed nothing urgent. No crisis demanded her immediate attention. No colleagues needed rescue.

And that's when panic truly took hold.

Her body physically needed stress hormones to function normally. Without them, she felt unmoored from reality. The absence of urgency left a vacuum where her purpose had been.

Useless. Irrelevant. Empty.
Her brain had operated in emergency mode for so long that normal stimulation felt like sensory deprivation. Now, deprived of her chemical lifeline, disintegration seemed imminent.

I don't know who I am without this.

And that realization terrified her more than any deadline ever could.

Parenting in the Pause

That afternoon, Rachel picked up Ethan from kindergarten, determination overriding discomfort.

Her phone remained silenced in her purse. No emails interrupted his excited chatter about playground adventures. No mental task list could compete with his stories.

For the first time in months, she was fully present—focus undivided, attention complete. And yet...

Wrongness lingered beneath the surface. Her fingers itched to check notifications. Her mind generated phantom emergencies requiring immediate attention. Her brain continued craving the stress chemicals it had come to depend on.

Even when she was doing the right thing, it didn't feel right.
This revelation illuminated the path ahead:

Burnout recovery couldn't be accomplished overnight. Breaking stress addiction required more than willpower. Her nervous system needed complete retraining.

This wasn't a simple mindset shift or motivational challenge. It was neurological rewiring—reconfiguring pathways carved by years of chronic stress.

The Crash That Always Comes

Evening descended, and with it, complete exhaustion unlike anything Rachel had experienced.

Not the satisfied tiredness following productive work. Not the pleasant fatigue after exercise.

This was cellular depletion—gravity multiplied, thinking fragmented, even simple decisions overwhelming. This bone-deep exhaustion made standing in the shower feel like running a marathon.

This wasn't restful tiredness. This was nervous system recalibration. This was her body fighting against years of biochemical conditioning.

She had spent years running on synthetic energy.

Now, without the chemical cocktail that kept her functioning, her body struggled to remember how to generate and conserve natural energy. The withdrawal symptoms weren't just psychological; they were physical evidence of a system in crisis.

The Science of Recovery Nobody Tells You

When Ethan finally fell asleep, Rachel texted Dr. Hughes from the darkness of her bedroom:

Rachel: *"Why do I feel WORSE now that I'm trying to slow down?"*

Dr. Hughes responded almost immediately:
Dr. Hughes: *"Because you're detoxing. And detox is never comfortable."*

Stress addiction operates beyond mindset—it's fundamentally biological.

Here's what was happening inside Rachel's brain:

Her dopamine-cortisol cycle was crashing.
Her neural pathways had formed deep associations between urgency and reward. Without that chemical pattern, motivation flatlined. Her brain, accustomed to emergency-level stimulation, interpreted normal environments as understimulating and potentially threatening.

Her nervous system interpreted calm as danger.
After years of high alert status, her body had forgotten how to recognize safety. Parasympathetic functions—rest, digestion, recovery—had atrophied from disuse. Now that she was attempting to slow down, her system interpreted the change as potential danger rather than relief.

Her brain was craving stress with addict-like intensity.
Just as caffeine withdrawal causes headaches and sugar withdrawal triggers intense cravings, stress withdrawal creates a constellation of symptoms: restlessness, irritability, exhaustion, brain fog, and a profound sense of loss.

This explains why most people relapse into burnout.

The discomfort deceives you into believing you need the very thing destroying you. Stress becomes both poison and antidote.

The only way through? Endure the withdrawal.

The Hardest Part of Letting Go

That night, Rachel lay awake, ceiling shadows shifting as hours passed.

Ethan slept peacefully down the hall. Her inbox contained nothing that couldn't wait until morning. The world continued spinning without her constant attention.

And yet...

Emptiness echoed where purpose once lived. The urge to create urgency—to generate a problem she could solve—pulled at her thoughts. Discomfort radiated through her body, making stillness feel like a form of punishment rather than relief.

Who am I if I'm not constantly putting out fires?

For years, stress hadn't just been her condition—it had been her identity.

She was the fixer who never failed, the problem solver everyone relied upon, and the high performer who thrived under conditions that crushed others.

But now, as she finally released her grip on chaos...

She realized she had no idea who existed beneath those roles.

Who Am I Without the Hustle?

Rachel had always known exactly who she was professionally.

The marketing executive with the golden touch. The crisis manager who never lost her cool. The woman who could transform impossible deadlines into accomplished realities.

But now?

Uncertainty clouded what once seemed crystal clear.

She had invested so many years chasing the next deadline, the next problem, the next opportunity to prove her value through sacrifice that she'd never stopped to ask:

What happens when I stop running?
Now, without a constant emergency to define her boundaries, she felt formless—a person without edges. The sensation terrified her more than any challenge she'd faced at Vertex.

Had stress been the adhesive holding her identity together?

The Fear of Slowing Down

Three days into her recovery, Rachel felt worse, not better. No overworking. No caffeine overload. No artificial urgency.

She should have experienced improvement—that's what wellness articles promised, what recovery platforms guaranteed.

She didn't.

Motivation evaporated like morning dew. Irritability simmered beneath every interaction. Emptiness expanded where purpose once lived.

Why do I feel like I'm failing when I'm finally taking care of myself?

Her brain, accustomed to operating in crisis mode, anxiously searched for threats to manage—creating psychological discomfort in their absence.

Without stress, she had forgotten how to function.

The Identity Crisis of Burnout Recovery

Popular wisdom suggests burnout recovery centers primarily on rest, meditation, and self-care rituals.

But Rachel confronted a more difficult truth:

Quitting stress isn't just about recovery. It's about reinvention.

She had built her entire sense of value on perpetual motion.

Being stressed signified importance—proof that her work mattered.

Being overworked represented dedication—evidence of her commitment.

Being needed gave her purpose—validation of her worth.

Without these external metrics...

Who was she?

This question haunted her quiet moments, more challenging than any work problem she'd ever faced.

The Mirror Moment
That evening, Rachel confronted her reflection in the bathroom mirror.

Exhaustion had left visible evidence—dark crescents beneath her eyes, tension lines around her mouth, a dullness in her complexion that expensive skincare couldn't disguise.

This was stress's signature, written across her face.

And yet...

I don't even know how to exist without it.

She had operated in survival mode for so long that peace felt like a foreign country—unknown, potentially dangerous, requiring a language she hadn't yet learned.

This explains why people relapse into burnout.

Not because they enjoy the damage. Not because they seek exhaustion. But because the familiar, even when harmful, feels safer than the unknown.

Rachel stood at a crossroads:
Cling to her stress-addicted self—the version she knew how to be. Step into uncertainty—and discover who she might become without chaos as her cornerstone.

For the first time, she understood the fundamental truth:
Burnout recovery wasn't just about quitting stress. It was about excavating the person buried beneath it.

Relearning How to Be Present

That night, Rachel sat beside Ethan on the living room sofa. No phone competed for her attention.

No laptop glowed nearby.

No distractions divided her focus.

Just mother and son in the quiet evening light.

Ethan glanced up at her, uncertainty clouding his expression.

"You're not working?"

Three words that pierced her heart more effectively than any criticism ever could.

He had already normalized her absence—expected it—even when she sat right beside him. She swallowed hard, forcing a smile. *"Nope. Just us tonight."*

Initially, wariness shadowed his features—as though he didn't quite trust this unexpected gift of presence.

But gradually...

His small body relaxed against hers. Stories poured from him—school adventures, dinosaur facts, playground politics—treasures he'd been storing up. The tension in his shoulders melted as he settled into the safety of her undivided attention.

Rachel felt something unfamiliar stir within her.

For the first time in years, she was fully present—and beneath the discomfort of withdrawal, it felt like coming home.

Perhaps this connection was what she'd been chasing all along.

The Hardest Part of Change

Rachel had initially conceptualized burnout recovery as primarily physical—rest, sleep, nutrition, and exercise.

But reality revealed a more complex challenge:
Recovery demanded breaking lifelong patterns that had become neural superhighways in her brain. It required unlearning stress as a core identity when her entire sense of self had been built upon it. It meant choosing an entirely different way of existing—even when that new path felt wrong, uncomfortable, and fundamentally threatening.

The hardest part of quitting stress isn't stopping.

It's learning how to live without it when your entire operating system was designed around its presence.

The Illusion of a Quick Fix

Rachel had assumed liberation would follow automatically once she stopped the harmful patterns.

She would feel immediate relief. Mental clarity would return naturally. Freedom would arrive like a gift once she put down her shackles.
Reality proved more complicated

Instead of liberation, she felt disoriented.

Work at Vertex felt strangely two-dimensional without the urgency that once gave it depth. Without constant pressure, her days felt structureless, shapeless. Life itself seemed emptier without the artificial intensity that had colored her experiences.

She had run so long and so hard that standing still felt like falling.

Why She Missed the Chaos

Her days had transformed beyond recognition.

Morning panic had been replaced with quiet intention. Impossible deadlines no longer dominated her calendar. Late nights chasing productivity had given way to reasonable hours and actual rest.

It should have felt liberating—the cage door finally opened. Instead?

It felt like loss.

She missed the adrenaline rush when solving impossible problems. She craved the validation that came with being everyone's emergency contact. She mourned the identity that came with being irreplaceable.

I thought I wanted peace, but now it just feels like I'm disappearing.

This explains why stress addiction persists despite its devastating cost.

Not because people can't identify the problem—but because they don't know what to replace it with.

Building a New Kind of Energy

After two weeks of struggle, Rachel realized a fundamental truth:

She couldn't simply subtract stress without adding something in its place.

She didn't just need less chaos—she needed a new source of vitality.

Redefining Productivity

For years, Rachel had measured success through metrics of quantity. Emails answered. Meetings attended. Problems solved. Fires extinguished. *But what if different measurements mattered more?*

The quality of her presence with Ethan. The depth of joy experienced in quiet moments. How well she tended to herself—not just her responsibilities.

This wasn't about working less.

It was about redirecting her exceptional capacity toward what truly mattered.

The False Starts

Breaking free from stress addiction didn't follow a linear path.

Some mornings, calm embraced her like an old friend. Other days, the craving for chaos returned with vengeance. Certain triggers—a particular email tone, a specific client request—still activated her stress response.

What if this grip never fully loosens?

Dr. Hughes had prepared her for this reality:

Recovery isn't linear. Discomfort will arise repeatedly. Setbacks don't indicate failure—they're integral to growth.

The goal isn't perfection but persistence.

What She Was Really Afraid Of

One evening, sitting in rare silence, Rachel confronted the truth beneath her struggle.

This journey wasn't just about quitting stress.

It was about abandoning a version of herself that only felt valuable through suffering.

Who would she be without the hustle?

Someone deserving of rest without guilt. Someone whose worth wasn't measured by exhaustion. Someone who could achieve remarkable things without sacrificing her health and relationships.

For the first time, she allowed herself to believe this might be possible—not just intellectually, but emotionally.

Choosing a New Reality

Rachel had operated under stress for years.

It had fueled her impressive career trajectory. It had defined her reputation for excellence. It had given her days structure and purpose. But standing at this crossroads, clarity emerged through the fog:

Stress had never been the source of her capability—it had been the thing limiting her potential.

She wasn't losing herself by abandoning chaos.

She was finally becoming who she was meant to be before the world taught her to equate suffering with success.

Breaking the Final Chain

The real test arrived unexpectedly on a Monday morning.

Her inbox overflowed with weekend accumulation. Her calendar displayed back-to-back commitments. A message from Vertex's CEO demanded immediate attention—a major campaign on the verge of collapse.

The old Rachel would have immediately shifted into emergency mode—heart racing, adrenaline surging, thoughts narrowing to crisis resolution.

She would have felt alive in the chaos.

But today?

She inhaled deeply, oxygen filling her lungs completely. Her shoulders relaxed deliberately away from her ears. A quiet voice within reminded her: *not everything is an emergency, even when it feels like one.*

This was the genuine breakthrough.

Not abandoning responsibility or escaping her career. Not pretending problems didn't exist. But choosing a fundamentally different relationship with pressure—engaging with challenges from a centered place rather than a frantic one.

She was reclaiming control of her nervous system.

The Redefinition of Success

Rachel had constructed her life around exhaustion—believing achievement required sacrifice, particularly of herself.

Now, gradually, she embraced a different definition of success:
Peace instead of perpetual panic. Clarity rather than constant chaos. Presence over relentless productivity.

This shift didn't diminish her ambition—it transformed it. She wasn't working less—she was working with greater intention. Her contributions at Vertex hadn't decreased—but the cost of making them had changed dramatically.

She hadn't lost her edge. She had finally found her center.

The Final Test: Trusting the Calm

A month passed.

The withdrawal symptoms had largely subsided. The compulsive urge to create urgency had loosened its grip. She experienced longer stretches where calm felt normal rather than threatening.

Then came the ultimate test.

A major client project. An aggressive timeline. Significant stakes for both Vertex and her career.

Every instinct in her body screamed to revert to old patterns.

I could work through the night. I could push myself beyond reasonable limits. I could surrender to the stress response—just this once.

But instead?

She established clear boundaries around the project scope. She worked with focused intensity rather than frantic energy. She protected her well-being without apologizing—recognizing that sustainable performance required sustainable practices.

For the first time, she navigated high-pressure circumstances without being consumed by them.

This wasn't just recovery. This was mastery.

The Moment She Knew She Was Free

Sunlight painted golden patterns across her balcony as Rachel watched the sunset, the city transitioning from day to evening beneath her.

No racing thoughts competed for her attention. No restless energy pushed her toward unnecessary action—just peaceful presence in the moment.

She closed her eyes, breathing deeply.

For years, she had pursued stress with addict-like devotion—believing it made her exceptional, valuable, worthy of respect and recognition.

But true strength existed elsewhere.

It lived in the stillness that allowed clear thinking when others panicked. It resided in the ability to maintain perspective under pressure. It flourished in the power to choose thoughtful responses rather than conditioned reactions.

She had reset her entire operating system.

And this time, there would be no returning to the harmful patterns that had nearly destroyed everything that mattered.

The New Rachel

Rachel still faced deadlines at Vertex, carried significant responsibilities, and encountered pressure in both her professional and personal spheres.

But now?
Stress no longer controlled her life. She controlled how she responded to it.

She had spent years believing stress was the fuel that powered her exceptional performance.

But the truth had revealed itself through her journey: **It was never fuel—it was a constraint limiting her true potential.**

And now? She had finally broken free from its chains.

What Comes Next? The Real Cost of Stress Addiction

As Rachel's personal transformation deepened, her perspective widened beyond her individual experience. Walking through Vertex's gleaming headquarters, she observed colleagues with newfound clarity—the dark circles beneath eyes, the tension in shoulders, the brittle laughter masking exhaustion.

She had escaped her personal addiction to stress. She had reclaimed her energy, her presence, and her authentic self from the jaws of burnout culture.

But as she watched talented people sacrificing themselves on the altar of productivity, a question formed:

How many others are caught in this same trap without recognizing it?

Her journey wasn't merely personal—it was part of something larger, more systemic. The stress addiction that had nearly destroyed her wasn't an individual failing. It was embedded in workplace expectations, relationship patterns, and cultural ideals that surrounded her everywhere.

And understanding the deeper system that kept people hooked on stress? That would become her next challenge.

For now, though, Rachel gathered her things and left the office at a reasonable hour. Ethan was waiting, and she would be fully present tonight for their dinosaur adventure.

Tomorrow would bring new challenges, but she would face them differently—not as an addict constantly chasing the next high, but as a woman who had discovered that real power comes not from the rush of stress, but from the strength to remain centered within it.

CHAPTER 2: THE BURNOUT BUSINESS MODEL

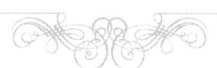

*Stress for Sale—How Corporations Turned
Your Burnout Into Billions*

The Trap You Never Saw Coming

Rachel Summers didn't wake up one day and decide to burn herself out.

The descent happened gradually, insidiously—like water dripping from a faucet into a basin, one drop at a time—until suddenly, she found herself drowning. By the time she noticed the rising tide, she was already gasping for air, her lungs burning with exhaustion.

Initially, she blamed herself, as high achievers often do.

Perhaps her time management skills needed refinement. Maybe she simply hadn't pushed hard enough through the fatigue. Possibly, she lacked the resilience that her more successful colleagues seemed to possess naturally.

But on a particularly gray Tuesday morning, as fluorescent lights buzzed overhead and she stared at her monitor, fingers hovering numbly over her keyboard, another email branded with that crimson *URGENT* flag appeared in her inbox. Something clicked into place—a moment of clarity cutting through the fog of exhaustion.

This wasn't just happening to her.

The evidence surrounded her in the open-plan office of Vertex Media. The hollow-eyed stares of colleagues. The constant parade of coffee cups. The nervous laughter that never quite reached tired eyes. The after-hours glow of computer screens illuminating faces that should have been home hours ago.

It was happening to everyone around her. And it wasn't accidental. It was methodical—calculated—planned.

Burnout wasn't a personal shortcoming or character flaw.
It was a business model, deliberately engineered and carefully maintained.

And for the first time, Rachel was about to discover just how deep the trap really went.

The Economy of Exhaustion

For years, Rachel had internalized the belief that burnout reflected her personal failure.

If only I managed my calendar better.
If only I developed more resilience.
If only I weren't somehow fundamentally flawed.

But today, as she sat at her ergonomically questionable desk, the room spinning slightly from a dangerous combination of caffeine overconsumption and chronic sleep deprivation, reality crystallized with startling clarity:

Burnout wasn't just her private struggle.

It was a systematic design.

Her gaze drifted across the landscape of Vertex's marketing department.

Sarah Chen, the brilliant graphic designer, is two cubicles down, massaging her temples with trembling fingers, fighting yet another stress-induced migraine—her third this month. David Kaplan, the normally cheerful content strategist, was now jittery and pale, and the recycling bin beside his desk was littered with empty energy drink cans before noon had even struck. Olivia Washington, who once radiated calm from her evening yoga practice, now hunched over her laptop well into the night, the glow of the screen highlighting dark circles beneath her once-bright eyes.

This wasn't some collective character defect.

This was a system functioning exactly as intended.

The Workplace That Fed on Stress

Rachel had navigated high-pressure work environments throughout her career at agencies and corporations, but only now did she recognize the deliberate pattern woven into the fabric of workplace culture.

Urgency wasn't an occasional necessity—it was the foundation of the business strategy.

She replayed last week's quarterly strategy meeting in her mind, words echoing with new significance.

The senior leadership team peppered their presentations with phrases like "thriving in a fast-paced environment" and "high performers excel under pressure." They publicly celebrated employees who pulled all-nighters to meet impossible deadlines, showcasing their exhaustion as a badge of honor. Meanwhile, those who protected their time and maintained boundaries were conspicuously absent from recognition, their contributions rendered invisible by their refusal to sacrifice themselves on the altar of artificial urgency.

This wasn't merely a toxic workplace culture that had evolved organically. It was a deliberate operational framework—a business model predicated on human depletion.

Rachel's role at Vertex wasn't simply to produce exceptional marketing campaigns.

It was to remain exhausted enough to never question the fundamental premise of the game she played.

The Manipulation of Meaning

Rachel had constructed elaborate justifications for her perpetual state of overwhelm.

Those emails marked URGENT carried the weight of a genuine emergency—surely lives hung in the balance. The cascade of back-to-back meetings signified her irreplaceable importance to the organization. The endless hours sacrificed to work represented proof that her contributions mattered in some cosmic calculation of worth.

But what if these were elaborate illusions, carefully crafted to exploit her need for purpose?

What if stress wasn't evidence of her value, but rather of her manipulation? With newfound skepticism, she pulled up an email chain from the previous week that had consumed an entire weekend of her life.

- *"We need this ASAP."*
- *"Can you jump on this now?"*
- *"Super urgent—drop everything else."*

Her heart rate accelerated as she scrolled through the messages, her body automatically responding to the remembered panic of the moment. She continued reading, searching for the catastrophic crisis that had justified her canceled plans with Ethan, her missed sleep, and her skipped meals.

It was a single misplaced comma in a presentation slide.

Nausea rolled through her stomach, the bitter taste of realization rising in her throat.

I abandoned my son's soccer game for this? I laid awake until 3 AM for this?

The revelation hit her with physical force: it had never been about the importance of the work itself.

It was about maintaining a state of perpetual overwhelm that prevented employees from recognizing the manipulation at play.

The Price of Being a 'Good Employee'

Rachel had dedicated years to embodying the ideal worker.

She arrived before sunrise, coffee in hand, ready to tackle yesterday's emergencies. She remained available around the clock, her phone never silenced, and her laptop was always within reach. She swallowed complaints about impossible workloads, wearing her stoicism as a professional asset.

And what had this dedication earned her?

Migraines that throbbed behind her eyes for days, resistant to medication. A sleep schedule so severely disrupted that even on rare quiet nights, her body refused to rest. A five-year-old son who had stopped asking the heartbreaking question, *"Mommy, will you be home for dinner tonight?"* because he'd learned through painful repetition that the answer was almost always no.

She had surrendered everything to Vertex Media. And the company had accepted every sacrifice without hesitation or acknowledgment.

The realization expanded beyond her personal situation to a broader question: How many thousands of people had traded their health, relationships, and joy for the illusion of security, believing this exchange was simply the cost of professional success?

Rachel's thoughts drifted to her father, his story suddenly relevant in ways she hadn't previously recognized.

He had devoted thirty years to a corporation that referred to employees as "family" in every town hall meeting—right until the moment they eliminated his position without warning or ceremony, leaving him adrift at fifty-seven with health issues developed during decades of stress and overwork.

Was her path really any different from his?

The Breaking Point

That evening, Rachel remained at her desk long after most had departed, fatigue penetrating to her marrow, bones feeling heavy beneath her skin.

A notification appeared on her screen. *URGENT: Need this ASAP.*

Her pulse accelerated automatically, the Pavlovian response to urgency so deeply ingrained that it bypassed conscious thought.

I should respond immediately. I should drop everything to address this crisis. I should demonstrate my reliability and commitment.

The familiar thoughts arose—and then, unexpectedly, a new one emerged:

No. No, I shouldn't.

She inhaled deeply, oxygen filling her lungs completely for what felt like the first time that day.

For the first time in her career at Vertex, she looked at the urgent message, recognized its manufactured nature, and made a different choice. Her hand moved to the laptop's edge—and closed it with quiet deliberation.

Her fingers trembled against the smooth surface, the small act of rebellion sending adrenaline coursing through her system.

It felt wrong, dangerous, forbidden.

Her mind screamed warnings: *They'll think you're not committed! They'll find someone more dedicated! They'll question your value!*

But her body registered something different—*a quiet recognition that this boundary, however small, felt right on a cellular level.*

She leaned back in her chair, heart pounding against her ribs, a curious mixture of terror and exhilaration flooding her system.

What happens if I stop participating in my own exploitation?

The answer remained unclear, the future suddenly unwritten. *But for the first time in years, she felt curious enough to find out.*

The System Fights Back

Rachel had always subscribed to the meritocratic narrative—that sufficient dedication would eventually yield proportional rewards.

A salary that reflected her true contribution. A title that granted genuine authority. Autonomy over how she structured her time and energy.

But the moment she took the first small steps away from complete subservience to the burnout machine, the system's response was swift and unmistakable.

- 📥 Two unanswered emails—reasonable given her focus on an actual priority project—transformed into "concerned" inquiries from her supervisor.

- 📌 A declined 9:00 PM meeting invitation resulted in a strategically placed comment in a team channel.

- 💬 "Rachel, is everything okay? You're usually the first to jump in and help."

The subtext was clear beneath the veneer of concern. Her years of proven excellence, her consistent results, her sacrifices for Vertex—none of it created a reservoir of goodwill. The moment she asserted the most minimal boundary, she became a problem requiring correction.

The Science of Why Burnout Is Profitable

As Rachel observed these dynamics with new awareness, the true nature of the game clarified in her mind.

Burnout isn't merely an unfortunate byproduct of modern work—it's a deliberate revenue strategy.

- 🔬 The neuroscience reveals why exhausted employees benefit corporate bottom lines:

> **Chronic stress keeps workers physiologically trapped in survival mode.**
>
> - Sustained elevated cortisol levels impair function in the **prefrontal cortex**—the brain region responsible for critical analysis, long-term planning, and complex decision-making.
> - The resulting cognitive impairment forces the brain to default to **reactive, short-term thinking** rather than strategic evaluation.

These neurological changes produce predictable, profitable outcomes:

Overwhelmed employees lack the cognitive bandwidth to question problematic workplace policies or practices. They conflate frenetic activity with meaningful productivity, working longer hours while accomplishing less of genuine value. Most insidiously, they develop dependency on the neurochemical cocktail of stress hormones, requiring the sensation of urgency to feel motivated and engaged.

The system doesn't benefit from employees operating at their full cognitive capacity—it profits from workers too depleted to recognize their own exploitation.

Rachel had been a prime example of this phenomenon.

Until today.

The First Consequence of Saying No

Rachel began testing small boundaries, treating them as experiments in reclaiming her autonomy.

She implemented a technology curfew, closing work applications after 8:00 PM. She evaluated meeting invitations critically, declining those where her presence added no genuine value. She carved out protected time for focused work rather than remaining perpetually responsive to others' demands.

Initially, these changes passed without comment, as though the system hadn't yet registered the small rebellions.

But then—subtly at first, then with unmistakable intention—the consequences materialized.

Her manager's previously effusive praise became notably absent during team meetings. Her name disappeared from the distribution list for a high-visibility project labeled "critical priority." A colleague made a seemingly casual remark within earshot: "Guess Rachel's finally decided to take it easy."

The substance of her work remained exemplary—nothing had changed except her refusal to sacrifice her well-being on the corporate altar.

And that deviation alone marked her as a potential threat to the established order.

The Loyalty Trap

Rachel's instinctive response to this subtle undermining was to prove them wrong through renewed self-sacrifice.

Work earlier, stay later, respond faster. Demonstrate through redoubled effort that her boundaries didn't diminish her value. Show them she remained dedicated despite her small acts of self-preservation.

But as this familiar impulse arose, a counterrealization struck with unexpected force:

Every burned-out employee is ultimately disposable.

Every overworked "family member" remains part of the corporate tribe only until their utility diminishes.

Every personal sacrifice made for organizational benefit evaporates from institutional memory the moment it becomes inconvenient to remember.

How many dedicated workers had given their health, their relationships, their very lives to organizations, only to discover their replaceability when they could no longer sustain the punishing pace?

She refused to become another statistic in this grim calculation.

The Scarcity Myth: Why You're Afraid to Walk Away

Rachel recognized that her struggle extended beyond the visible culture of Vertex Media.

She was battling something more fundamental: the neurobiological wiring of her own brain.

🔬 **The perception of scarcity triggers primitive survival mechanisms:**

- When we perceive potential loss—whether of income, professional identity, or organizational belonging—the brain responds by **flooding the body with stress hormones.**
- This biochemical reaction creates a **threat response disproportionate to reality,** causing people to remain in harmful situations because the brain interprets change as more dangerous than continued suffering.

This neurological response explains why so many remain tethered to toxic work environments:

Fear of financial instability overrides concern about physical and mental deterioration. Cognitive biases lead to minimizing genuine harm with rationalizations like "everyone deals with stress."

Limited perspective creates the illusion that better alternatives don't exist.

Rachel had remained trapped in this mindset for years, her perception narrowed by stress and fear.

But what if the scarcity narrative was fundamentally false?

What if other organizations valued sustainable performance?

What if success could be achieved without self-destruction?

What if paths existed that didn't require surrendering her health and relationships? She inhaled deeply, expanding her lungs against the constraint of habitual anxiety. *I don't have to participate in a system designed to deplete me.*

The Decision That Changed Everything

One particularly chaotic Tuesday morning, Rachel's inbox exploded with urgent messages.

📩 A client crisis. A departmental error. A deadline unexpectedly accelerated.

Just weeks ago, her response would have been automatic—caffeine-fueled determination to solve everything immediately, regardless of the personal cost. Her former self would have canceled lunch, worked through the evening, and measured her value by her capacity to absorb organizational chaos.

The Rachel who sat at her desk today paused before reacting, asking questions her previous self would have considered heretical:

Does this situation genuinely require my immediate intervention?

Is this an authentic emergency, or merely the latest iteration of manufactured urgency? Will substantive harm result if I address this in two hours rather than two minutes?

The entire burnout economy depends on employees never asking these fundamental questions.

With deliberate movement, she closed her email application and rose from her desk, walking toward the small kitchen area for a glass of water and a moment of reflection.

Let others manage the latest "crisis."

And as cool water slid down her throat, an unfamiliar sensation expanded through her chest—something she hadn't experienced in her professional life for longer than she could remember:

Agency.

The Backlash

Rachel had anticipated that choosing sustainability over stress would feel primarily liberating.

And briefly—it did.

She had set a reasonable boundary instead of surrendering to artificial panic.

She had stepped away from orchestrated urgency rather than being consumed by it. She had prioritized genuine productivity over performing the theater of busyness.

But organizational systems don't surrender control without resistance. The workplace that had benefited from her stress addiction didn't simply accept her emerging boundaries.

The following morning, subtle changes permeated her professional interactions.
The typically friendly tone in team communications carried a noticeable chill. Her supervisor's usual warm acknowledgments were replaced with businesslike brevity. A strategy session occurred after hours—her absence noted but her input neither requested nor missed.

She had transitioned from "indispensable asset" to "potential liability" seemingly overnight.

The Psychology of Punishment

Why do organizations respond this way to boundaries?

> Because burnout culture **requires universal participation to maintain its power**.
>
> If employees recognize overworking as a choice rather than a necessity, they **might begin opting out en masse**. If one individual successfully breaks free from the cycle without consequence, **others might follow their example**.

> If healthy boundaries become normalized within the culture, **the entire exploitative framework risks collapse.**
>
> *Rather than examining the system itself, the organization redirects attention to the individual who dares question it.*

And despite her intellectual understanding of these dynamics, Rachel remained vulnerable to their emotional impact.

Have I irreparably damaged my professional standing?

Have I sabotaged the career I've worked so hard to build? Have I made a catastrophic miscalculation?

The engineered doubt functioned precisely as designed—creating uncertainty and fear to drive compliance.

The Subtle Ways They Pull You Back

With growing awareness, Rachel observed the sophisticated mechanisms Vertex employed to recapture those attempting to escape stress addiction:

📧 The superficially casual "check-in" messages

💬 "Not sure if this slipped through the cracks, but..."

The communications artfully designed to trigger guilt

💬 "I ended up finishing this at midnight—hope you had a good evening."

The strategic exclusion from significant conversations

💬 "We made that decision yesterday evening—assumed you wouldn't want to be bothered after hours."

The tactics rarely involved direct confrontation—instead, they created a subtle current constantly pulling her back toward unhealthy patterns, *suggesting her absence created burdens for others and diminished her professional relevance.*

For a brief, unguarded moment? The manipulation nearly succeeded.

The Dopamine Trap

🔬 **The neurochemical basis for this compulsion was clear:**

> Because her brain had developed dependence on specific reward pathways.
>
> The stress of urgency triggers dopamine release. The anticipation of checking messages creates a dopamine release. The sensation of being needed generates dopamine release.
>
> She wasn't merely habituated to overwork—she was neurochemically tethered to the reward system it provided, a system as real and powerful as any substance dependency.

Now that she'd begun interrupting these patterns, her brain demanded the neurochemical rewards it had come to expect.

She closed her eyes, inhaling deeply through her nose, feeling the expansion of her ribs beneath her shirt.

Nothing catastrophic will happen if I don't check. The world will continue turning without my immediate attention.

For the first time in recent memory, she stepped away from the laptop without yielding to the compulsion, choosing instead to make a cup of tea and read a novel that had sat untouched on her nightstand for months.

The Power Shift

The following morning, Rachel implemented a change that would have seemed inconceivable mere weeks earlier.

She left her phone on silent through breakfast with Ethan. She prepared for the day thoughtfully, without the familiar rush of checking messages between tasks. She entered the Vertex Media building at a reasonable hour, walking rather than running to her desk.

The office environment hadn't changed in any visible way—the same ergonomic chairs, the same fluorescent lighting, the same background hum of conversation and typing. Yet her experience within that space had fundamentally transformed—not because the external had shifted, but because her internal relationship to it had.

She no longer reacted to every stimulus like an extension of the system. She chose her responses consciously.

And in that momentous shift from reaction to choice, a profound truth crystallized in her awareness:

The burnout business model only functions when we willingly participate in it.

The Realization That Changed Everything

For years, Rachel had operated under a series of professionally damaging misconceptions:

That extreme effort correlated directly with professional value.

That immediate responsiveness equated to indispensability.

That visible exhaustion represented the price of admission to meaningful success.

But each of these beliefs crumbled under scrutiny.

The organization's most influential individuals weren't those working longest hours—but those who maintained calm amid chaos.

The highest compensated weren't those handling the most tasks—but those focusing on the most consequential ones.

The most respected weren't those visibly sacrificing themselves—but those delivering exceptional results without drama or martyrdom.

As this understanding settled into her awareness, a decision crystallized:

I refuse to continue equating my worth with my willingness to self-destruct.

From this moment forward, she would engage with work from an entirely different paradigm.

Redefining Work Without Stress

Rachel had invested her entire professional identity in a particular vision of achievement.

First to arrive at the office, demonstrating commitment through early-morning dedication. Last to leave each evening, her car often alone in the parking garage under darkening skies. Unfailingly agreeable regardless of the toll each new demand extracted.

But as she observed her colleagues from her new perspective—watching them scramble frantically in response to the latest "urgent" directive from leadership—the theater of it all became painfully apparent:

Burnout wasn't the inevitable companion of excellence—it was evidence of a successfully implemented manipulation.

She would no longer participate in her own exploitation.

But if stress wasn't the engine of achievement, what would replace it?

The question loomed large, unfamiliar territory stretching before her.

And the uncertainty filled her with both apprehension and unexpected possibility.

The Fear of Doing Less

Rachel began declining unnecessary meetings with deliberate intentionality.

The first refusal generated intense guilt, her body physically reacting with tension and discomfort.

The second triggered anxiety, her mind generating catastrophic scenarios about potential repercussions.

By the third, something unexpected emerged—a quiet sense of empowerment, territory reclaimed from the wilderness of obligations.

But deeply ingrained patterns resist change, sending their roots into the foundations of identity.

One afternoon, a message from her supervisor appeared:

 "Hey Rachel, can you jump on a quick call? Just need your input on something."

Experience had taught her that "quick calls" invariably expanded to consume whatever time she allocated and more.

Should I just agree to maintain goodwill?

Will declining damage my professional reputation?
Will asserting boundaries mark me as uncooperative?

Her cursor blinked in the empty response field as conflicting impulses battled within her.

Then, with surprising steadiness, she typed a response that would have been unthinkable months earlier.

She wrote: *"I'm deep in focused work right now. Can this wait until tomorrow morning? If it's truly urgent, I can review a summary of the key points."* Her finger hovered over the send button momentarily before pressing it decisively.

Her hands trembled slightly, autonomic nervous system responding to perceived threat.

What if the response is negative? What if this crosses an invisible line?

 Reply: "No problem at all. I'll send you notes this afternoon and we can connect tomorrow."

Rachel stared at the screen, momentarily puzzled by the anticlimactic response.

That was the entirety of the reaction? No pushback? No passive-aggressive undertone?
As the implication settled, a startling recognition emerged:

Much of the pressure she'd experienced throughout her career had originated not from external demands but from her own internalized expectations.

The Productivity Lie

Throughout her professional life, Rachel had measured her contribution through quantitative metrics.

Tasks completed. Emails processed. Hours invested.

 Yet research consistently demonstrated the opposite relationship:

- ☑ **Deep work**—extended periods of uninterrupted focus—produces **exponentially superior outcomes compared to fragmented attention.**
- ☑ **Task-switching** and multitasking reduce cognitive performance by **as much as 40% through attention residue.**
- ☑ **Strategic work limitation** consistently generates higher quality output than endless grinding.

The most effective professionals weren't necessarily the visibly busiest—they were those who protected their focus with fierce intention.

Rachel had been caught in a tragic paradox: doing more while accomplishing less of genuine significance.

That pattern ended today.

The Scarcity Myth: What If I Miss Out?

As Rachel implemented her boundaries, her colleagues remained entrenched in the stress economy.

Checking messages during dinner with families. Joining conference calls during vacations. Responding to non-emergencies with emergency-level urgency.

Despite her intellectual commitment to change, she felt the gravitational pull of their collective behavior.

What critical developments might I miss during my offline hours?
Will my influence diminish if I'm not constantly present?

Am I sacrificing opportunity by refusing to remain perpetually available?

These questions represented scarcity psychology functioning exactly as designed.

🔬 **The evolutionary basis for this fear response:**

> The human brain evolved in environments where social exclusion represented existential threat. In prehistoric contexts, separation from the tribe often meant death. This ancient wiring manifests in modern workplaces as fear of professional irrelevance or replacement—a threat that feels primal and overwhelming despite its modern context.

This explains why intelligent professionals remain in harmful work situations—the primitive brain perceives the potential loss of status or belonging as more dangerous than the actual damage of chronic stress.

But what if this perception of scarcity was fundamentally inaccurate?

The Shift That Changed Everything

Rachel made a foundational decision that altered everything that followed:

She would evaluate success through fundamentally different criteria.

She would establish her own rhythm rather than allowing external demands to dictate her pace.

She would systematically retrain her stress response to distinguish between genuine emergencies and manufactured urgency.

This philosophy manifested in immediate practical application when an email marked "URGENT ACTION REQUIRED" appeared in her inbox.

Rather than triggering her usual immediate response, she deliberately closed the notification.

No instant reaction. No stress-induced focus shift. No guilt about temporary non-responsiveness.

When she returned to the message an hour later after completing her priority task?

 The situation had resolved itself without her intervention.

How much of her stress had been generated by phantom emergencies rather than genuine crises?

The realization expanded through her awareness like ripples across still water:

She had been complicit in creating her own burnout—and now, she possessed the power to dismantle it.

When You Stop Playing the Game, the Game Pushes Back

Over several weeks, Rachel accumulated small victories against burnout's dominion.

She discerned which urgencies required attention and which would evaporate without intervention. She protected time for substantive, focused work rather than remaining perpetually reactive. She established clear boundaries between professional and personal domains.

For the first time since joining Vertex, she experienced genuine agency—work became something she controlled rather than something that controlled her.

But systems designed to exploit rarely surrender their advantage without resistance.

And now, the pushback intensified beyond subtle cues to unmistakable pressure.

The Pressure of the Crowd

Rachel had anticipated resistance from leadership as her primary challenge. Reality proved more complex and insidious.

- 📌 The most persistent pressure came from unexpected sources—her peers.

- 💬 "Must be nice to have the luxury of 'focus time' while the rest of us handle the real emergencies."

- 💬 "So should we just assume you're unavailable after 6:00 now, or...?"

- 💬 "Remember when we could count on you to step up when things got tough?"

The collegial atmosphere had subtly soured. Her image transformed from respected team member to potential liability. Her boundaries were reframed as selfishness, forcing others to compensate for her new limitations.

And nothing generates more potent social pressure than watching someone escape a system in which others remain trapped.

The Social Conditioning of Overwork

 The psychological dynamics underlying this response were predictable:

> Burnout culture persists through both organizational design and social enforcement.
>
> Humans naturally calibrate behavior to match group norms.
>
> When collective behavior normalizes overwork, deviation creates cognitive dissonance. Those unable or unwilling to assert similar boundaries often respond with hostility rather than inspiration.

Rachel wasn't merely changing her individual work patterns.

She was implicitly challenging the premise that everyone else's sacrifice was necessary.

And that representation of alternative possibilities threatened the justifications others had constructed for their own suffering.

The Sabotage Begins

Rachel had previously noticed subtle punishment for her boundaries, but the organizational response escalated to unmistakable intentionality.

She found herself systematically excluded from strategic conversations where her expertise would previously have been essential. High-visibility projects that aligned perfectly with her skills were assigned to others without explanation. Meeting schedules were established without consideration for her availability, and her absence was noted with pointed emphasis.

The message was being communicated with increasing clarity: return to compliance or face diminishing relevance.

The Rachel of six months ago would have interpreted these signals as directives to work harder, stay later, and prove her dedication through renewed self-sacrifice.

But what if she refused to read from that familiar script?

What if she released her attachment to approval from a system designed to exploit her?

She inhaled deeply, shoulders relaxing away from her ears.

I no longer need to demonstrate my value through my capacity for suffering.

Let the consequences unfold as they will.

The Almost-Relapse

The true test arrived unexpectedly on a Wednesday afternoon.

 "Rachel, we have a genuine emergency with the Northstar campaign. Need your immediate attention. Can you handle this ASAP?"

The message came directly from Elena Michaels, the Chief Marketing Officer—a rare direct communication from leadership that signaled genuine significance.

Her nervous system responded instantly to the stimulus.

> The perception of true urgency triggered dopamine release.
>
> The opportunity to solve a high-stakes problem promised satisfaction. The direct request from senior leadership offered validation.

Just this one time. This seems legitimately important. I don't want to damage my standing with executive leadership.

Her fingers moved toward the keyboard, ready to fall back into familiar patterns of reactive stress response.

Addiction doesn't disappear with awareness—it waits patiently for moments of vulnerability.

And this particular moment presented the perfect conditions for relapse.

The Pause That Saved Her

With conscious effort, Rachel interrupted the automatic response pattern.

She placed her palms flat on her desk. She closed her eyes briefly, focusing on the sensation of breath moving through her body. She allowed herself to experience the discomfort of resisting the conditioned urge.

This moment represents the critical juncture between habitual reaction and intentional response.

Instead of immediately sacrificing her current priorities, she evaluated the situation through new criteria:

Is this genuinely urgent, or merely presented as urgent to ensure immediate action? Would meaningful harm result from a thoughtful, measured response rather than an immediate reaction? What reasonable boundaries can I maintain while still contributing effectively?

Having considered these questions, she crafted her response.

She typed:
💬 "I understand the importance of the Northstar situation. I can dedicate focused attention to this, but I'll need until tomorrow morning to properly transition my current priority project and approach this with

full focus. If that timeline doesn't work, please let me know what specific elements need immediate attention, and I'll prioritize accordingly."

No unconditional surrender to external demands. No abandonment of her current commitments.

No sacrifice of her wellbeing for artificial urgency.

This represented the genuine transformation—not merely setting boundaries in theory, but maintaining them under authentic pressure.

The Shift in Power

Rachel anticipated significant negative consequences for her measured response to executive urgency.

Perhaps a direct reprimand. Perhaps thinly veiled threats about team commitment. Perhaps damage to her professional standing.
Instead, something entirely unexpected occurred.

> Reply from Elena: "That works fine. Tomorrow morning is soon enough. Thanks for the quick response."

The simplicity of the acceptance momentarily disoriented her, expectations of conflict unfulfilled.

Had the anticipated negative consequences existed primarily in her imagination?

The implication expanded in her awareness, reshaping her understanding of workplace dynamics:

Much of the urgency she'd responded to throughout her career had been artificial. Much of the pressure she'd experienced had been self-imposed. The system maintained power largely through employees' internalized beliefs rather than actual enforcement.

The recognition shifted something fundamental in her relationship with work.

When Stress Isn't Running the Show

Rachel had operated in perpetual reaction mode for the entirety of her professional life.

Responding instantaneously to notifications regardless of their importance. Abandoning current tasks for any new request labeled urgent. Measuring her professional worth by her capacity to absorb chaos without complaint.

But now?

She had reclaimed agency over her attention and energy.

And the organization that had previously benefited from her stress addiction now faced the unfamiliar challenge of relating to her as a self-directed professional rather than an exploitable resource.

The Shock of Stability

Four weeks had passed since Rachel began dismantling her participation in the burnout economy.

She no longer checked emails during dinner with Ethan.

She maintained clear technological boundaries between work and personal time. She evaluated urgency claims critically rather than responding automatically.

Initially, the change felt disconcerting—as though she were somehow failing to fulfill unwritten professional obligations.

But as weeks passed?

Her thinking became sharper, connections between concepts emerging with newfound clarity. Her physical well-being improved, the constant headaches and tension gradually subsiding. She experienced genuine presence in non-work moments, the mental weight of perpetual preoccupation lifting from her consciousness.

Burnout had convinced her that stress functioned as essential fuel for performance. But without it? She discovered capabilities previously obscured by chronic depletion.

The Response from Work

Rachel had prepared herself for escalating organizational resistance.

Perhaps her supervisor would begin systematically reducing her responsibilities.

Perhaps colleagues would increasingly exclude her from important conversations. Perhaps subtle penalties would accumulate into career stagnation.

But something entirely unexpected emerged instead.

✉ Email from the Director of Talent Development: "Several team members have noted your improved productivity and work life boundaries. Would you be willing to share some of your time management approaches with the department?"

Rather than facing rejection for her boundaries, she encountered curiosity about them.

She had anticipated punishment for her deviation from burnout norms. Instead, she had become an object of observation—and potentially, emulation.

She wasn't suffering professional damage as feared.

She was pioneering an alternative approach that others secretly wished to follow.

The Recalibration Phase

Despite her progress, Rachel's body continued adjusting to its new operating conditions.

🔬 Breaking neurochemical dependency isn't instantaneous.

Initially, her brain continued searching for urgency-based stimulation, manufactured emergencies that would trigger familiar chemical responses. Certain evenings, the compulsion to check work communications remained powerful, a phantom limb of her former patterns. Her nervous system occasionally generated anxiety in response to reasonable workloads, conditioned to interpret normalcy as insufficient.

During these moments, she reminded herself of the fundamental distinction she now understood:

💬 **Stress serves as a tool for specific situations—not as a chronic operating condition.**

And she refused to allow it to reclaim its position as her primary energetic source.

Redefining Success

Rachel had previously evaluated her professional performance through metrics that ensured perpetual inadequacy:

- ☒ Quantity of output regardless of significance.
- ☒ Problems addressed regardless of whether they required her specific expertise.
- ☒ Exhaustion level as validation of effort invested.

Now, she measured success through fundamentally different criteria:

- ☑ Quality and impact of **focused, high-value work** completed without distraction.
- ☑ Level of **mental presence** maintained during both professional and personal interactions.
- ☑ Effectiveness in **protecting and directing her energy** toward genuinely consequential activities.

The transformation extended beyond merely surviving her career.

She was creating a sustainable approach to meaningful achievement.

The Personal Side of Recovery

The changes extended far beyond her professional life, rippling through every domain of her existence.

She attended Ethan's school events without checking her phone beneath the table. She reconnected with Emily and other friends she'd neglected during years of work absorption. She rediscovered activities that had once brought her joy—reading fiction, weekend hiking, and cooking meals that didn't come from delivery services.

One evening, as she sat on the edge of Ethan's bed during their nightly dinosaur story ritual, he looked up at her with an expression of wonder that tightened her throat.

💬 *"You're different now, Mommy."*

The simple observation carried more emotional weight than any professional recognition she'd ever received.

This represented what burnout had stolen most cruelly—irreplaceable moments of connection that no corporate achievement could possibly compensate for.

She refused to surrender another day to a system designed to consume her from the inside out.

The Final Test: Can She Sustain This?

Rachel had transformed her relationship with work.

But the external environment remained largely unchanged.

The burnout business model would continue attempting to recapture her participation. Old patterns would occasionally whisper seductive rationalizations for returning to familiar stress addiction. Genuine pressure would inevitably arise, testing her new boundaries and perspectives.

Yet something fundamental had shifted within her:

> She no longer needed external validation through visible overwork to recognize her intrinsic value.

And that internal recalibration? It represented her true liberation from the burnout economy.

What Comes Next? Breaking the Dopamine-Cortisol Cycle

Rachel had discovered that burnout wasn't merely an unfortunate professional habit—it was a biochemical addiction methodically cultivated by workplace systems benefiting from employee depletion.

As she observed her colleagues still trapped in stress cycles, a new question emerged:

> If burnout functions as genuine addiction, what neurological mechanisms maintain its grip on otherwise intelligent professionals?

She recognized that her journey toward sustainable performance required more than surface-level boundary setting.

She needed to understand the invisible neurochemical forces that had maintained her compliance in a system designed to exploit her.

The dopamine rewards that made urgent emails feel irresistibly important. The cortisol surges created the illusion of productivity while systematically damaging her health. The neurochemical cocktail that transformed stress from an occasional useful response into a chronic addiction.

Dismantling the business model of burnout represented only the beginning of her journey. Understanding and recalibrating the brain chemistry that enabled it? That challenge lay immediately ahead—the next frontier in her ongoing liberation from a system designed to consume her one stress response at a time.

As Rachel closed her laptop at a reasonable hour and prepared to leave the office, she noticed several colleagues still hunched over their desks, faces illuminated by screen glow, coffee cups long empty beside them. For the first time, she didn't see dedication in their postures—she recognized fellow addicts caught in a cycle they didn't yet understand.

Tomorrow would bring new challenges. But she would face them differently—not as reactive crises demanding her immediate sacrifice, but as manageable situations to be addressed with calm intention by a professional who finally understood the true nature of the game.

CHAPTER 3: THE DOPAMINE-CORTISOL TRAP

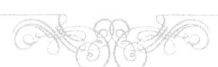

*Why Rest Feels Like Withdrawal—
The Hidden Neuroscience of Why You
Can't Relax*

What If Calm Feels Worse Than Chaos?

Rachel Summers had been certain that escaping the burnout cycle would bring immediate relief.

Logic dictated that removing stress would naturally result in a cascade of positive effects. Her mind would quiet, her body would relax, and the constant tension between her shoulder blades would finally release its grip.

But reality told a different story.

Instead of the anticipated peace, a strange restlessness crawled beneath her skin. Even when no deadlines loomed, her thoughts scattered in a dozen directions. The quiet moments she'd fought so hard to create now filled her with an inexplicable anxiety that tightened her chest and quickened her breath.

She found herself instinctively searching for problems to solve, challenges to overcome, fires to extinguish—as though her nervous system couldn't tolerate the absence of emergency.

The question formed as she stared at her untouched phone one evening, a realization dawning that disturbed her more than any work crisis:

Why do I feel more lost now than when I was drowning in work? Why does rest feel like failure rather than recovery?

Sunlight slanted through her apartment window, illuminating dust particles floating in the air. Rachel watched them drift, a perfect metaphor for her scattered thoughts. The stillness that should have been comforting instead felt fundamentally wrong, as though she'd failed some essential test of worthiness.

She had spent years running on the chemical high of constant urgency. Now that the artificial stimulation had been removed, her body and mind were rebelling against the unfamiliar calm, demanding the neurochemical cocktail they had come to depend on.

That's when the truth crystallized with startling clarity—burnout wasn't simply a bad habit she had developed. It was a full-fledged biochemical addiction her body had come to require for normal functioning.

Emily Notices Before Rachel Does

"Your leg isn't bouncing," Emily Whitaker observed, green eyes narrowing with scientific interest over the rim of her coffee cup.

The late afternoon sun filtered through the café's window, casting golden light across the small table separating the two women. They had been best friends since college—long before Rachel's gradual descent into stress addiction had begun reshaping her personality and habits.

Emily, a clinical psychologist specializing in workplace trauma, had watched the transformation happen in real time—Rachel's healthy ambition slowly morphing into something more compulsive, more desperate, more consuming.

"What do you mean?" Rachel asked, genuinely confused.

Emily gestured toward Rachel's legs with her mug. "You always bounce your right leg when we're sitting. Always. For the past three years, at least. It's your tell—how I know your mind is already back at work even when your body is here."

Rachel glanced down, suddenly aware of the stillness in her limbs. "That's... weird."

"Not weird." Emily tilted her head, professional curiosity evident beneath her casual tone.

"Different. Interesting. When was the last time you checked your phone?"

The question caught Rachel off-guard. She couldn't remember—had it been an hour? Two? Her hand didn't even twitch toward her bag, where her phone remained silent and forgotten.

"Hours ago," she admitted, the realization striking her as both foreign and vaguely unsettling.

Emily's expression softened, a subtle smile playing at the corners of her mouth. "That's new for you."

The observation wasn't delivered as criticism but as a clinical notation—a scientist documenting an unexpected change in a long-established pattern. Emily had seen Rachel at her worst: checking emails during birthday celebrations, disappearing to take calls during dinners, her attention perpetually fragmented by the digital tether to work.

Rachel shifted uncomfortably in her chair, suddenly aware of how deeply she had normalized her own dysfunction. She had been so thoroughly immersed in survival mode that she hadn't recognized how unnatural "normal" had become—how alien genuine peace now felt in her body.

The Science of Stress Addiction

📖 **The conversation with Emily unearthed memories of an earlier discussion with Dr. Alexander Hughes months before.**

When she'd first consulted him about her exhaustion, Rachel had dismissed his warnings as overly dramatic. She had nodded politely while inwardly rolling her eyes, certain that burnout was simply a matter of being tired—a condition easily remedied with a weekend of self-care, perhaps a massage or a recreational yoga class.

Dr. Hughes's office came back to her now—the comfortable leather chair, the soft lighting, the certificates on the wall identifying him as one of the country's leading neuropsychologists specializing in high-performance burnout. His gentle voice had delivered uncomfortable truths she wasn't ready to hear.

She had been profoundly wrong about the nature of her condition.

Dr. Hughes had explained the neurochemistry in careful detail:

Dopamine & Cortisol: Partners in a Destructive Dance

Dopamine — The Chase Chemical
The neurochemical that drives motivation wasn't designed for constant stimulation. In our ancestral environment, dopamine surges came from meaningful achievements and survival necessities. In the modern workplace, it's hijacked by endless notifications, artificial deadlines, and the perpetual "almost there" of never-ending task lists.

This chemical fuels anticipation and pursuit—the sensation of being on the verge of accomplishing something significant. It creates the rush of checking items off a list, of being needed, of solving problems under pressure.

Most insidiously, dopamine makes stress feel good—transforming urgency into a reward rather than a warning signal.

Cortisol — The Stress Hormone
Evolution designed cortisol as an emergency response, not a chronic condition. It triggers the fight-or-flight response, flooding the body with glucose, increasing heart rate, and sharpening focus temporarily.

When constantly elevated, cortisol keeps the body in a state of physiological emergency, burning through resources meant to be conserved. It creates a sense of alertness that feels productive but systematically damages cognitive function over time.

Most dangerously, sustained cortisol exposure desensitizes the brain to normal stress levels. Like any addictive substance, the dosage must continually increase—which is why Rachel eventually needed higher stakes and greater pressure just to feel engaged with her work.

The cycle operated with devastating efficiency: The more stress Rachel experienced, the more her brain adapted to require it. Her neural pathways were rewired to interpret calm as threatening rather than safe. She had neurologically conditioned herself to function only under conditions of perceived emergency.

This explained why high-achievers so often struggle with basic relaxation.

They don't merely choose stress or have difficulty "switching off"—their physiology has literally adapted to require the chemical cocktail of urgency to feel normal.

The First Symptoms of Withdrawal

Rachel leaned forward, elbows on the café table, massaging her temples where a dull pressure had been building all afternoon. The coffee before her had grown cold, forgotten during their conversation.

"So why do I feel worse now that I'm doing everything right?" she asked, frustration evident in her voice. "I'm setting boundaries. I'm not checking emails after hours. I'm leaving work at a reasonable time. Shouldn't I feel better?"

Emily added a splash of oat milk to her second cup of coffee, considering her response. As both a friend and a psychologist, she walked a delicate line between professional insight and personal support.

"Because your body thinks something's wrong," she said simply. "You've been running a physiological marathon for years. Now that you've stopped sprinting, your system is crashing—not because stopping is bad, but because your biochemistry doesn't know how to function without the stress chemicals it's adapted to."

Rachel had spent years operating on artificial energy. Now that the chemical supply had been reduced, her system was experiencing predictable withdrawal effects.

🔥 **Dr. Hughes had methodically outlined this recovery phase during their sessions:**

Phase 1: The Cortisol Crash
When cortisol suddenly drops after chronic elevation, the body experiences symptoms similar to coming off stimulants. Energy levels plummet beyond normal tiredness into profound fatigue. The nervous system, accustomed to operating in emergency mode, struggles to function under normal conditions.

Phase 2: The Dopamine Deficit
Without the constant dopamine hits from urgency, problem-solving, and crisis management, the reward pathways in the brain register a chemical deficit. This creates a pervasive sense of flatness—activities that should be pleasurable feel empty, motivation wanes, and an unsettling emotional numbness develops.

Phase 3: The Anxiety Backlash
Perhaps most counterintuitively, the nervous system often misinterprets the absence of stress as a danger signal rather than relief. Having adapted to chronically elevated threat levels, normal conditions register as suspiciously quiet—prompting the brain to begin manufacturing concerns and seeking problems where none exist, simply to return to its accustomed state of hypervigilance.

Rachel wasn't merely changing habits or adjusting her schedule. She was undergoing neurochemical withdrawal from substances her own body had been producing in harmful quantities for years.

Dr. Hughes' Plan: Retraining Rachel's Brain

Sunlight streamed through the floor-to-ceiling windows of Dr. Hughes's office, illuminating the space with natural light that contrasted with the fluorescent environment of Vertex Media. Rachel sat in the comfortable leather chair, legs crossed, fingers interlaced in her lap.

"So... I'm literally addicted to stress?" she asked, the clinical framing both validating her struggle and slightly horrifying in its implications.

Dr. Hughes nodded, his expression compassionate but matter-of-fact. At fifty-seven, with silver threading through his dark hair and decades of experience treating high-performing professionals, he projected a calm confidence that made even uncomfortable truths feel manageable.

"Yes. But the good news is, we can systematically address this. Your brain learned these patterns, which means it can unlearn them with the right approach."

He outlined a comprehensive strategy, each element designed to address different aspects of stress addiction:

Step 1: Nervous System Reset
- ☑ **Structured recovery periods** — Not passive rest, but intentional practices that activate the parasympathetic nervous system. Daily sessions of 30 minutes minimum dedicated to breathwork, cold exposure therapy, or slow, mindful movement practices.
- ☑ **Circadian rhythm restoration** — Regular exposure to natural light, particularly morning sunlight, to regulate cortisol's natural daily cycle rather than keeping it artificially elevated.

Step 2: Dopamine Detox & Recalibration
- ☑ **Elimination of artificial dopamine triggers** — Temporarily removing or strictly limiting social media scrolling, news consumption, and unnecessary multitasking that provide small but constant dopamine hits.
- ☑ **Focus on deep work rather than reactive tasks** — Prioritizing extended periods of uninterrupted focus on meaningful projects rather than the quick hits of solving minor problems or responding to non-urgent messages.
- ☑ **Intentional natural dopamine stimulation** — Daily engagement with activities that generate healthy dopamine responses: physical exercise, genuine social connection, music, or creative pursuits.

> **Step 3: Cognitive Reframing**
> ☑ **Distinguishing between urgency and importance** — Developing new mental filters to accurately categorize tasks based on genuine priority rather than emotional response or external pressure.

Dr. Hughes explained that this wasn't merely a psychological exercise but a complete neurological reprogramming—one that would ultimately allow her to experience greater productivity and clearer thinking without the damaging effects of chronic stress activation.

When Rest Feels Like Failure

Two weeks into Dr. Hughes' protocol, Rachel sat alone in her apartment, practicing what he called "intentional stillness"—thirty minutes of doing absolutely nothing productive. No reading. No television. No planning. Just sitting with herself and observing her thoughts without acting on them.

It was excruciating.

Her body physically rebelled against the inactivity. An uncomfortable energy buzzed beneath her skin. Her mind generated an endless stream of tasks she should be completing, problems she should be solving, and emails she should be answering.

More distressing than the physical discomfort was the emotional response—a profound sense of worthlessness that expanded with each passing minute of "unproductivity." The stillness didn't feel peaceful or restorative. It felt like failure, like waste, like evidence of some fundamental inadequacy.

Rachel had always assumed that stress was something external that happened to her—a condition imposed by circumstances beyond her control.

Now she faced a more uncomfortable truth: her nervous system had adapted to interpret calm as threatening and stress as normal.

The absence of urgency wasn't registering as relief but as danger—a physiological alarm signaling that something was wrong precisely because nothing was wrong.

Dr. Hughes had warned her about exactly this phase of recovery.

"Your body will fight you," he had explained. "It's like an immune response to change. The discomfort isn't evidence that you're doing something wrong—it's confirmation that you're disrupting patterns that need to be disrupted."

The insight provided little comfort as she sat in her living room, watching sunlight move across the wall, feeling simultaneously restless and exhausted, her body chemistry desperately seeking the familiar stress response it had come to depend on.

Why Does Doing Nothing Feel So Wrong?

Fourteen days into her recovery protocol, Rachel met Emily at their regular café, the familiar environment highlighting how differently she experienced herself within it.

She had diligently followed Dr. Hughes' recommendations: limiting artificial stimulation, engaging in daily nervous system regulation practices, prioritizing deep work over reactive tasks. The objective measures showed improvement—better sleep, reduced physical tension, fewer stress-related headaches.

Yet subjectively, she felt strangely disconnected from herself, as though operating in an unfamiliar body.

"It's like I don't know who I am when I'm not running around putting out fires," she admitted, absently stirring her tea. "I should feel better, but instead I feel... I don't know. Lost?"

Emily considered her friend thoughtfully. The afternoon light highlighted the subtle changes in Rachel's appearance—less tension around her eyes and improved color in her complexion, even as uncertainty clouded her expression.

"That's because you've been defining your worth by how much you could handle for years," Emily observed. "Your entire sense of self has been built around being the person who manages impossible workloads, solves unsolvable problems, achieves the unachievable."

The observation struck with uncomfortable precision. Rachel exhaled slowly, recognizing the truth in it.

"When you remove that measuring stick, it's disorienting," Emily continued gently. "It's not just a chemical addiction—though that's real. It's an identity addiction. You're not just withdrawing from stress hormones. You're withdrawing from the story you've been telling yourself about who you are and what makes you valuable."

That was it exactly. Rachel wasn't merely breaking dependency on biochemical patterns—she was dismantling a fundamental belief about her worth as a person. The realization simultaneously terrified and liberated her.

She wasn't just addicted to stress—she was addicted to being needed, to being the indispensable problem-solver, to constant external validation of her value.

The "Competence Trap" — Why High-Achievers Stay Stuck

During their next session, Dr. Hughes elaborated on what Emily had intuited:

"You're experiencing what we call the 'Competence Trap,'" he explained, sketching a simple diagram on his notepad. "It's particularly common among high-achievers and perfectionists."

The trap operated in a self-reinforcing cycle:

> Some individuals develop stress addiction through the biochemical dopamine-cortisol pathway. Others—like Rachel—become addicted primarily because their entire self-concept becomes entangled with their capacity to handle pressure.

The Competence Trap's Mechanics:
- Throughout her career, Rachel had received consistent positive reinforcement—promotions, recognition, respect—specifically for handling crises, working beyond reasonable hours, and "saving the day" when others couldn't.
- This external validation became internalized, creating a core belief that her value derived from her capacity to endure more pressure than others.
- When stress was removed from the equation, so was the primary source of her sense of professional worth and personal identity.
- Without constant challenges to overcome, she experienced not relief but a profound identity threat—a fear of becoming irrelevant, unremarkable, or replaceable.

"This explains why many exceptionally capable professionals resist delegation, boundary-setting, or reasonable workloads," Dr. Hughes noted. "It's not just workaholism or perfectionism in the traditional sense. It's that their entire self-concept is built around being the most reliable, most capable person in any room."

Rachel nodded slowly, the explanation resonating on a visceral level.

"I don't think I know how to exist without constantly proving myself," she admitted, the vulnerability of the statement catching in her throat.

"That," Dr. Hughes replied gently, "is the real withdrawal you're experiencing. You're not just detoxing from cortisol and dopamine—you're detoxing from external validation as your primary source of self-worth."

The First Breakthrough: Learning to Rest Without Guilt

Among Dr. Hughes' many challenging prescriptions, one had seemed particularly absurd to Rachel initially:

"Spend one hour each day doing absolutely nothing productive. No multitasking. No background stimulation. Just sit with yourself in the present moment."

When first assigned, the directive struck her as impossible—a waste of precious time she could use for "actual recovery," like exercise or sleep. She nodded politely while internally dismissing the suggestion as therapeutic overkill.

But after three weeks of limited progress, she reluctantly committed to trying it.

The first attempt lasted only fifteen minutes before anxiety compelled her to check her phone. The second attempt stretched to twenty minutes before she invented an urgent task requiring immediate attention. By the third day, physical discomfort—restless legs, racing thoughts, a tightness in her chest—made sitting still nearly unbearable.

Her mind generated a constant stream of objections and escape routes:

What if I'm missing something important? What if I could be using this time more efficiently? What if this whole exercise is just making me fall further behind?

Then, on the fifth day, something shifted.

Twenty-seven minutes into the practice, a subtle change occurred. The constant internal chatter didn't disappear, but it seemed to recede slightly, as though moving from the foreground to the background of her awareness. For brief moments, she experienced the sensation of simply existing without needing to justify that existence through productivity.

For years, Rachel had outsourced her sense of worth entirely to external metrics—tasks completed, problems solved, recognition earned. She had forgotten how to value herself apart from what she accomplished.

Now, sitting alone in her living room as afternoon light filtered through curtains, she glimpsed something she had lost long ago—the radical notion that her humanity had inherent value independent of her output.

The revelation wasn't dramatic or emotional. It arrived quietly, a simple thought that nonetheless shifted something fundamental in her perception:

Perhaps I don't need to earn the right to exist through constant achievement.

Emily's Perspective: The Friend Who Knew the Old Rachel

Emily observed Rachel's transformation with the unique perspective of someone who had known her before stress had reshaped her personality and habits.

She remembered the Rachel from graduate school—ambitious but balanced, driven but present, capable of genuine engagement with life beyond work. She had witnessed the gradual shift as Rachel climbed through professional ranks: the increasing preoccupation with status, the growing inability to be fully present, the subtle replacement of joy with accomplishment as life's primary currency.

Emily saw how profoundly difficult this recovery process was for her friend—not just the physiological withdrawal, but the existential recalibration it demanded. She watched Rachel struggle to accept that her value wasn't diminished when she wasn't constantly proving herself through overwork and self-sacrifice.

She had waited years for Rachel to recognize what was happening—to understand that she was trading irreplaceable life moments for the temporary high of professional validation.

Now that Rachel was finally changing, Emily felt both hopeful and cautious. Recovery wasn't linear, and the pull of old patterns remained powerful.

During a quiet dinner at Rachel's apartment, Emily finally voiced her thoughts.

"I like this version of you," she said simply, reaching for her water glass. "The one who actually finishes a meal without checking her phone.

The one who seems present rather than just physically here."

Rachel looked up from her plate, a flash of vulnerability crossing her features.

"But I don't think you fully trust her yet," Emily added gently.

Rachel sighed, shoulders relaxing with the exhale.

"I'm working on it," she admitted. "Some days I feel like I'm making progress. Other days I feel like I'm failing at recovery the same way I used to feel like I was failing at work—never quite enough."

Emily nodded, understanding the paradox. The most challenging aspect of Rachel's transformation wasn't just learning new habits—it was learning to trust that she was intrinsically enough, even when she wasn't in constant motion, proving her worth to herself and others.

Can You Handle Success Without Stress?

Rachel had built her entire professional identity on a fundamental assumption: stress made her better.

She had convinced herself that stress kept her sharp, that adrenaline improved her performance, and that pressure brought out her best qualities. Deadlines weren't just organizational necessities but catalysts for her success. The sensation of urgency hadn't registered as a warning but as motivation—the feeling of being fully engaged, fully alive.

Now, operating without her familiar chemical cocktail of stress hormones, a terrifying question emerged:

If stress wasn't actually the source of her capabilities or the foundation of her success...

What was?

The question contained both threat and promise. If she could succeed without self-destruction, what justified the years she had spent sacrificing her well-being?

Conversely, if her abilities remained intact—or even improved—without chronic stress, what possibilities might open before her?

The First Real Test: A Work Crisis Without Overload

The genuine test of her transformation arrived unexpectedly on a Tuesday afternoon.

Rachel sat at her desk reviewing quarterly projections when the notification appeared on her screen—an email from Elena Michaels, Vertex's Chief Marketing Officer, with a subject line that would have sent her into immediate panic mode just months earlier:

Subject: Last-Minute Presentation—Need Your Help ASAP

The message detailed a situation requiring immediate attention: a critical client presentation scheduled for the following morning had encountered significant problems. The team needed her expertise on short notice.

Pre-recovery, Rachel would have responded instantly, dropping all current priorities. She would have canceled her evening plans without hesitation, worked through the night if necessary, sacrificed sleep, meals, and personal boundaries to "save the day." The resulting exhaustion would have been worn as a badge of honor—evidence of her exceptional dedication and indispensability.

Rachel felt the familiar biochemical response begin—the quickening pulse, the narrowing focus, the surge of adrenaline preparing her for emergency response mode.

This time, however, she recognized the reaction for what it was—a conditioned pattern, not an inevitable response.

She took three deep breaths, feeling the air fill her lungs completely before exhaling slowly. She assessed the situation objectively rather than emotionally, distinguishing between genuine urgency and manufactured emergency.

"I'll handle this," she told herself calmly. "But I won't burn myself out doing it."

For the first time in her career, she approached a crisis with the radical notion that delivering exceptional work and maintaining her well-being weren't mutually exclusive goals.

Dr. Hughes Explains the Final Phase of Recovery

During their scheduled session that Friday, Rachel described the presentation crisis and her response to it with a mixture of pride and lingering uncertainty.

"I handled it well," she explained, sitting in her usual chair in Dr. Hughes' office. "I addressed the situation effectively, delegated appropriately, maintained boundaries, and still delivered exceptional work. The client was thrilled with the presentation."

Dr. Hughes nodded, recognizing the significance of this milestone.

"But something still feels... off," Rachel continued, struggling to articulate the subtle disconnection she experienced. "Even with this success, I don't quite feel like myself. It's as though I'm operating in someone else's life—doing all the right things but not fully inhabiting them."

Dr. Hughes leaned back slightly, his expression thoughtful.

"That's because you're still waiting for stress to return and define you," he observed. "You're handling situations differently but haven't yet fully integrated these changes into your identity. You're operating from new behaviors but still carrying old expectations."

The insight struck Rachel with unexpected force. She had indeed been approaching recovery as a temporary state—a phase to move through before returning to some modified version of her former self.

"Recovery isn't just about changing what you do," Dr. Hughes continued. "It's about transforming how you see yourself. Right now, you're in the liminal space between identities—you've left behind the stress-addicted achiever, but you haven't fully embraced who you're becoming instead."

Rachel nodded slowly, recognizing the truth in his assessment. The discomfort she experienced wasn't evidence of failure but of transformation—the natural disorientation that comes with fundamental change.

"I need a new way to measure success," she acknowledged quietly.

How High Performers Redefine Success

Dr. Hughes outlined the three phases of genuine recovery from stress addiction, explaining that Rachel was entering the final and most transformative stage:

Phase 1: Breaking the Stress Addiction
- ☑ Developing the ability to distinguish between genuine importance and manufactured urgency.
- ☑ Recognizing that calm isn't an enemy to be feared but a resource to be cultivated.
- ☑ Retraining neural pathways to function effectively without requiring crisis as motivation.

Phase 2: Learning to Operate from Stability Instead of Adrenaline
- ☑ Building the capacity for sustained attention without needing external pressure.
- ☑ Handling genuine challenges without resorting to self-destructive patterns.
- ☑ Maintaining productivity through focused intention rather than reactive urgency.

Phase 3: Finding Fulfillment Beyond Work
- ☑ Developing an identity that exists independently of professional accomplishments or external validation.

- ☑ Discovering genuine satisfaction in moments of presence rather than exclusively through achievement.
- ☑ Cultivating the ability to trust success that comes without suffering as its prerequisite.

"You've made remarkable progress through the first two phases," Dr. Hughes noted. "You've broken the physiological addiction to stress hormones, and you've demonstrated that you can perform at a high level without self-sabotage."

Rachel had indeed navigated the most visibly challenging aspects of recovery—the uncomfortable withdrawal symptoms, the rebuilding of focus without crisis as motivation, the development of new work patterns that didn't require constant adrenaline.

"But now comes the deeper work," he continued. "Recalibrating your understanding of who you are when accomplishment isn't your primary source of worth and identity."

This final phase wouldn't be measured by external metrics or behavioral changes, but by an internal shift in how she experienced herself and her place in the world—a transformation that couldn't be rushed or forced, only cultivated through consistent practice and compassionate awareness.

The Biochemical Price of Modern Productivity

The contemporary workplace doesn't reward genuine efficiency—it rewards visible effort and performative exhaustion.

Working longer hours earns more recognition than producing better results in less time. Constant availability is valued above focused, high-quality contribution. The appearance of struggling under pressure often garners more acknowledgment than calm competence.

But this paradigm doesn't reflect true productivity—it perpetuates a destructive addiction while creating the illusion of necessity.

The human brain evolved in environments where stress was an occasional, life-saving response to genuine threats—not a chronic operating condition. Yet millions of professionals now exist in a perpetual state of physiological emergency, their nervous systems never fully returning to baseline before the next perceived crisis activates them again.

And like any addiction, the longer the cycle continues, the more difficult normal functioning becomes without the stimulus—creating the deceptive impression that stress is essential rather than harmful.

How The Dopamine-Cortisol Loop Rewires Your Brain

Dr. Hughes explained that chronic stress creates not just psychological patterns but physical alterations in brain structure and function.

1. Dopamine Flooding — The Chase Mechanism

Dopamine, often mischaracterized as the "pleasure chemical," actually mediates motivation, anticipation, and pursuit. It's not about the reward itself but about the expectation of reward—the neurochemical that keeps us hunting, seeking, pursuing.

The modern workplace engineers constant dopamine triggers through artificial deadlines, immediate feedback loops, and performance metrics that keep employees perpetually chasing the next target, the next achievement, the next recognition.

The fundamental problem: Dopamine evolved to motivate pursuit, not satisfaction.

- The neurochemical surge comes while working toward a goal, not upon achieving it.
- This creates a hedonic treadmill where accomplishment provides only fleeting satisfaction before the next pursuit begins.
- Over time, this trains the brain to value the chase itself—the stress of pursuit—rather than the completion of meaningful work.

2. Cortisol Overload — The Stress Hormone's Hijack

Cortisol serves an essential function when properly regulated—preparing the body for effective response to genuine threats by increasing glucose availability, accelerating heart rate, and sharpening immediate focus.

But sustained elevation creates a cascade of harmful effects, impairing everything from immune function to cognitive processing. Most notably, it physically alters brain structure—shrinking the prefrontal cortex responsible for executive function while enlarging the amygdala that processes fear and emotional reactivity.

The resulting neural transformation: The more stressed you become, the less access you have to your highest cognitive capabilities—creating a vicious cycle where impaired decision-making creates more stress, further impairing function.

3. Adrenal System Burnout — The Energy Crash

The human body cannot sustain emergency-level hormonal output indefinitely. Eventually, the endocrine system responsible for producing stress hormones becomes dysregulated, leading to a constellation of symptoms:

- ☑ Crushing fatigue that rest doesn't resolve
- ☑ Cognitive impairment affecting memory and concentration
- ☑ Hypersensitivity to minor stressors
- ☑ Emotional flatness and detachment

Together, these neurochemical patterns create a self-perpetuating system where professionals simultaneously feel compelled to pursue constant productivity while experiencing diminishing returns in both satisfaction and capability.

Why High Achievers Struggle to Quit Stress

The most insidious aspect of stress addiction is that it masquerades as virtue—a necessary commitment to excellence rather than a destructive pattern requiring intervention.

High performers frequently rationalize their condition:

"I deliver my best work under pressure."

"A little stress keeps me motivated and engaged."

"If I don't maintain this pace, someone else will surpass me."

But these justifications represent adaptive responses to dysfunction—not evidence of optimal performance.

🔬 **Dr. Hughes explained how stress creates cognitive distortions that perpetuate its grip on otherwise intelligent individuals:**

1. Stress Creates an Illusion of Enhanced Energy
Cortisol stimulates the sympathetic nervous system, creating a sensation similar to a caffeine boost or second wind. This temporary enhancement of alertness is misinterpreted as sustainable energy.

The reality? This isn't genuine energy but a stress-induced override of normal fatigue signals—like removing the warning light rather than addressing the depleted fuel tank.

When the inevitable crash arrives, energy reserves are more depleted than if the warning signals had been heeded initially.

2. Busyness Becomes Confused with Effectiveness
In stress-addicted environments, visible activity—attending numerous meetings, responding instantly to communications, managing multiple simultaneous tasks—becomes the primary measure of contribution rather than meaningful outcomes.

This creates a perverse incentive system where appearing busy takes precedence over producing quality work. The constant context-switching and interrupted attention that results from this approach actively prevents the deep, focused thinking where genuine innovation and excellence emerge.

Neuroscience demonstrates conclusively that the highest-quality cognitive work happens during periods of sustained attention with minimal cortisol activation—precisely the opposite conditions from those cultivated in most high-pressure workplaces.

3. **The Withdrawal Period Creates a False Negative Signal**
When someone begins reducing stress after chronic exposure, they don't experience immediate relief but rather uncomfortable withdrawal symptoms—decreased motivation, emotional flatness, restlessness, and even temporary cognitive fog.

These transitional effects are misinterpreted as evidence that stress is necessary for functioning rather than recognized as the natural detoxification process of a system recalibrating to healthier operation.

This misinterpretation drives many back into stress addiction, convinced their performance decline confirms they "need" pressure to function optimally.

Professionals remain tethered to stress not because they enjoy suffering, but because their neurochemistry has been conditioned to require it for normal functioning—and the initial discomfort of breaking this dependency reinforces the illusion of its necessity.

Reversing the Damage: How to Break Free from the Trap

Liberation from the dopamine-cortisol cycle doesn't require eliminating stress entirely—a completely stress-free existence is neither possible nor desirable. The goal is to establish neural pathways that can engage with appropriate stress productively without becoming addicted to or dependent upon it.

🔬 Dr. Hughes provided Rachel with a comprehensive framework for rewiring her brain toward sustainable high performance:

Phase 1: Rebuild the Nervous System
☑ **Transition out of chronic sympathetic dominance** using specific techniques that activate the parasympathetic "rest and digest" system—strategic cold exposure, structured breathwork patterns, and intentionally slow movement practices that signal safety to the nervous system.

- ☑ **Systematically reduce artificial stimulation** by creating boundaries around news consumption, notification management, and digital task-switching that keeps the brain in a perpetual state of low-grade alarm.
- ☑ **Deliberately activate parasympathetic recovery** through practices that have been scientifically validated to lower cortisol—specific forms of nature exposure, single-tasking rather than multitasking, and targeted rest periods strategically placed throughout the day.

Phase 2: Redefine Dopamine Triggers
- ☑ Gradually replace artificial dopamine sources (social media, constant email checking, unnecessary notifications) with extended periods of deep work that generate more sustainable satisfaction.
- ☑ **Cultivate delayed gratification capacity** by structuring work around meaningful completion rather than constant partial attention—training the brain to associate dopamine release with genuine achievement rather than the illusory "busy" state.
- ☑ **Increase natural, sustainable dopamine pathways** through regular physical movement (especially in natural settings), daily exposure to morning sunlight, which regulates both dopamine and circadian rhythms, and engagement with activities that create flow states where time seems to disappear.

Phase 3: Rewire the Brain's Relationship with Productivity
- ☑ Develop new metrics for evaluating work beyond urgency or quantity—prioritizing impact and meaning over volume or speed.
- ☑ **Build tolerance for non-stimulation** through regular periods of healthy boredom—allowing the brain to reset dopamine sensitivity rather than requiring constant novel input.
- ☑ Transform the fundamental motivation source from stress-based reactivity to values-aligned intention—connecting work to deeper purpose rather than external pressure.

True exceptional performance isn't about functioning effectively despite stress—it's about cultivating the conditions where your highest capabilities can emerge without requiring the destructive effects of chronic stress hormones.

What Happens When You Stop Relying on Stress?

Rachel had progressed through each stage of the stress addiction cycle:

She had constructed her entire identity around her capacity to handle overwhelming pressures.

She had used stress as her primary motivational fuel for so long she'd forgotten alternatives existed.

She had systematically confused urgency with importance, activity with achievement.

And now?

She was discovering how to maintain exceptional performance without the biochemical dependency that had nearly destroyed her health, relationships, and joy.

She approached workplace challenges with a strategic focus rather than reactive panic. She maintained motivation through purpose and interest rather than artificial urgency. She had begun dismantling the false equation between self-sacrifice and professional value.

This represented the genuine transformation—not merely managing stress better, but fundamentally redefining what success felt like in her body and mind.

Final Thought: High Performance Without Burnout

For most of her professional life, Rachel had accepted without question the cultural mythology that stress functioned as rocket fuel for achievement.

But the scientific reality directly contradicted this narrative. Burnout isn't the inevitable companion of ambition but rather evidence of a fundamentally flawed approach to work. The most consistently exceptional performers aren't those who endure the most pressure, but those who master the allocation of their energy, attention, and recovery.

The dopamine-cortisol trap wasn't a necessary condition for achievement but a sophisticated mechanism designed to extract maximum effort with minimum awareness.

Liberation didn't require abandoning ambition or excellence—it demanded rejecting the false premise that suffering serves as a prerequisite for success.

The true measure of professional capacity isn't how much stress you can endure without breaking—it's how much clarity and effectiveness you can maintain regardless of external conditions.

Rachel wasn't simply recovering from burnout—she was pioneering a fundamentally different relationship with achievement, one that didn't demand her destruction as the price of her success.

What Comes Next? The Hidden Cost of Running on Empty

As Rachel integrated these neurochemical insights into her daily life, establishing new patterns and dismantling old dependencies, she noticed something unexpected—a question arising from her increasing stability:

> 💬 *Why do some days still leave me feeling deeply depleted, even when I'v maintained healthy boundaries and avoided stress triggers?*

The persistent fatigue puzzled her. She had expected that breaking her stress addiction would restore her energy completely. While she had experienced significant improvement, something still felt missing from her recovery equation.

She was beginning to recognize that stress hadn't merely hijacked her brain chemistry—it had been systematically depleting a more fundamental resource all along: her core energy reserves.

During their next session, she posed this question to Dr. Hughes, who nodded with recognition.

"You've addressed the neurochemical addiction," he explained, "but there's another dimension to burnout recovery we haven't fully explored yet—the energy depletion pattern that stress creates over time. Your body isn't just recovering from chemical dependency; it's rebuilding energy systems that have been operating in deficit for years."

Understanding how chronic stress had compromised her most essential physiological resources—and how to systematically restore them—represented the next frontier in her recovery journey.

As spring sunshine streamed through her office window the following Monday, Rachel closed her laptop at a reasonable hour, gathered her things, and left the building while daylight still illuminated the city streets. A text from Emily confirmed their dinner plans, and she felt a gentle anticipation for the evening ahead—a normal human pleasure that once would have been overshadowed by work preoccupations.

The dopamine-cortisol cycle no longer determined her experience of life. She had begun reclaiming her biochemistry from a system designed to exploit it—not by rejecting achievement or ambition, but by discovering that her greatest capabilities emerged precisely when she refused to sacrifice herself for the illusion of productivity.

Tomorrow would bring new challenges. But for the first time in years, she would meet them as a whole person—her nervous system regulated, her brain chemistry rebalanced, her identity expanding beyond the narrow confines of what she could accomplish under pressure.

The real journey was just beginning.

PART II:

THE HIDDEN COSTS OF ADDICTION

CHAPTER 4: YOUR STOLEN ENERGY

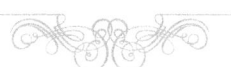

Stolen Life—The Silent Energy Drains Killing Your Vitality

The Silent Drain

Rachel Summers had conquered the most visible enemies of well-being.

Work hours had been tamed into reasonable boundaries. Her calendar now contained white space rather than back-to-back commitments. Artificial urgency no longer dictated her responses. By every conventional measure of burnout recovery, she was succeeding.

And yet, exhaustion clung to her like a second skin.

This wasn't the familiar fatigue that followed long hours at Vertex—the kind that a good night's sleep might remedy. This was something more pervasive, a bone-deep weariness that persisted despite adequate rest, proper nutrition, and reasonable workloads.

Standing at her kitchen counter one morning, sunlight slanting through the blinds as she waited for her coffee to brew, Rachel faced an uncomfortable question: If overwork wasn't depleting her anymore, what was?

It wasn't the late nights she had eliminated.

It wasn't the deadlines she had placed in proper perspective.

It wasn't even the workplace culture she had learned to navigate differently.

It was everything else.

The realization settled over her with surprising clarity. Throughout her recovery journey, she had meticulously protected her time—creating boundaries, rebuilding routines, reclaiming hours previously surrendered to Vertex Media.

But something essential had escaped her attention until now: No one had taught her how to protect her energy.

Why You're Always Running on Empty

Rachel had operated under a seemingly logical assumption: reduce the hours spent working, and vitality would naturally return. A mathematical equation where subtracting labor would automatically yield increased energy, mental clarity, and emotional presence.

Weeks into her transformed relationship with work, this fundamental premise revealed itself as incomplete at best, misleading at worst. Sitting in Dr. Hughes' office, afternoon light casting gentle shadows across his desk, she articulated the persistent puzzle.

"I'm doing everything right," she explained, frustration evident in her voice. "I've cut back my hours. I'm leaving work at a reasonable time. I've stopped checking emails at night." She gestured vaguely toward the world outside the window. "So why do I still feel like I'm perpetually running on fumes?"

Dr. Hughes nodded, unsurprised by the question. "Because you've addressed the most obvious drain, but not the most pervasive one."

He leaned forward slightly. "Your exhaustion was never just about your job, Rachel. That was simply the most visible manifestation of a much broader pattern."

The truth landed with uncomfortable precision: Her mental bandwidth—attention, willpower, and cognitive resources—was being steadily depleted throughout each day through dozens of seemingly inconsequential interactions with the modern world.

Overwork had merely been the final straw breaking an already overburdened system.

The Invisible Drains on Your Energy

🔬 "Why do people feel exhausted even when they're not engaged in conventionally 'difficult' work?" Dr. Hughes posed the question rhetorically, rising from his chair to sketch a simple diagram on his whiteboard.

"Because the human brain wasn't designed for the environment we've constructed around it," he continued, drawing circles representing different categories of energy depletion.

1. Digital Fatigue: Your Brain Wasn't Built for This Many Inputs

The first circle expanded as he labeled it.

> "Every notification, email alert, and social media update triggers what's called an 'orienting response' in your brain," he explained. "It's a survival mechanism designed to interrupt current activity and redirect attention toward potential threats or opportunities. Useful when those interruptions were rare—catastrophic when they occur hundreds of times daily."

He tapped the whiteboard with his marker.

> "Research from Stanford University demonstrates that constantly switching between tasks depletes cognitive resources at approximately twice the rate of sustained focus. Each transition demands neural reconfiguration, and that process consumes glucose and oxygen at accelerated rates."

2. Decision Overload: Every Choice Costs You Mental Energy

A second circle joined the first.

> "The prefrontal cortex—responsible for decision-making, impulse control, and planning—operates like a muscle. It fatigues with repeated use and requires recovery periods," Dr. Hughes continued. "Yet modern life demands hundreds of decisions daily, from trivial to significant."

Rachel nodded, recognizing her own experience in his words.

> "What should I eat? Which email deserves priority? Should I respond to this message now or later? Is this meeting worth attending? Each individual decision seems manageable, but collectively, they silently deplete the same finite resource that powers willpower, creative thinking, and emotional regulation."

3. The Dopamine Crash: How Mindless Scrolling Leaves You Tired

A third circle completed the triad.

> "Your brain's reward system evolved to motivate behaviors that supported survival—finding food, securing shelter, building social connections. Today, that same system is systematically hijacked by technologies designed to capture and monetize attention."

He gestured toward Rachel's phone resting on the edge of his desk.

> "Social media, news feeds, and even email provide irregular but frequent dopamine rewards—creating the neurological equivalent of slot machines. These platforms trigger brief chemical surges that feel momentarily energizing but leave neurotransmitter systems depleted afterward. The brain substitutes the illusion of productivity for genuine accomplishment, leaving you mentally exhausted without equivalent satisfaction."

Rachel absorbed this information, connecting theoretical concepts with her lived experience. She had eliminated excessive work hours, but these invisible energy thieves continued operating unimpeded, extracting cognitive resources throughout her day.

"So I've stopped working myself into exhaustion," she summarized, "but I haven't stopped the world from steadily draining my energy in a thousand small ways."

Dr. Hughes nodded, returning to his chair. "Exactly. Which means your next challenge isn't just about what you remove from your life—it's about redesigning how you engage with everything that remains."

Rachel straightened slightly in her chair, the beginning of determination replacing resignation.

"Then I'm taking it back," she said simply.

The 24-Hour Experiment: Cutting the Drains

The following morning, Rachel stood in her kitchen, contemplating the experiment she'd designed for herself. The plan was simple but radical: for one complete day, she would systematically eliminate the major energy leaks Dr. Hughes had identified.

No notifications would interrupt her focus.

No mindless scrolling would hijack her attention.

No unnecessary decisions would deplete her mental resources.

She had mapped out the day carefully, identifying likely challenges and planning specific alternatives for habitual behaviors. Still, an undercurrent of anxiety accompanied her resolve—a recognition that she was about to challenge patterns far more ingrained than she had previously acknowledged.

"It's just 24 hours," she reminded herself, filling her water bottle while pointedly ignoring her phone charging on the counter. "I'm going to discover what happens when I stop feeding the distractions that have been feeding on me."

The metaphor struck her as particularly apt. These invisible energy thieves hadn't merely been taking her attention—they had been consuming her vitality while providing just enough intermittent reward to mask the transaction.

Today, that exchange would stop.

Hour 1: The Pull of Distraction

The first test came immediately. Rather than reaching for her phone upon waking—her invariable morning routine for years—Rachel had deliberately placed it across the room, charging.

The physical discomfort that followed surprised her. A distinct sensation of unease spread through her body, a craving as identifiable as hunger or thirst. Her brain protested the deviation from its expected stimulation with remarkable intensity.

Her mind generated compelling justifications:

What if something important happened overnight?
What if someone needs to reach me?
What if I'm missing crucial information?

She sat on the edge of her bed, observing her thoughts rather than immediately acting on them. The urge to check her phone wasn't merely a habit—it was a conditioned response that bordered on compulsion.

"How much of my focus has been stolen before my day even begins?" she wondered aloud, the question resonating in her quiet bedroom.

The realization was both illuminating and disturbing: She had never truly understood how deeply she'd been programmed to seek constant input, how thoroughly her attention had been commodified without her conscious participation.

This wasn't merely a behavioral pattern but something more profound—a dependency on persistent stimulation that began the moment consciousness returned each morning.

Hour 3: The Withdrawal Hits

By mid-morning, seated at her desk at Vertex Media, Rachel encountered the full force of attention withdrawal.

Her workspace had been deliberately reconfigured. Her phone was placed in a drawer, the email application was closed, and notifications were disabled across all platforms. A single project occupied her screen—deep, focused work that required sustained attention rather than reactive responses.

Her neurological rebellion intensified.

Restlessness manifested physically—her leg bouncing unconsciously, fingers drumming against the desk edge. Her thoughts scattered like startled birds, refusing to land on the task before her. The compulsion to "just check" something—anything—crescendoed until it dominated her awareness.

Dr. Hughes had warned her about this phase. "What you'll experience isn't just inconvenience or boredom," he had explained. "It's genuine withdrawal. Your brain has adapted to constant novel stimulation. When that input suddenly stops, your neurochemistry protests the change."

The physiological parallels were undeniable. Just as the body develops dependency on substances that artificially manipulate its chemical balance, her brain had developed dependency on the dopamine hits triggered by digital interruptions and task-switching.

Her nervous system had been trained to operate in a perpetual state of partial attention—never deeply focused, never fully at rest, always scanning for the next bit of novel information.

Rachel closed her eyes briefly, acknowledging the discomfort without surrendering to it. "I'm not just tired," she reminded herself. "I'm overstimulated, and I'm finally breaking the cycle."

Hour 6: Clarity Returns

Something shifted as the day progressed toward noon. The transition wasn't dramatic but unmistakable—like fog gradually lifting from a landscape, revealing details previously obscured.

Rachel noticed it first in her thinking, which seemed to flow with unexpected fluidity. Complex concepts connected more readily.

Decision-making required less effort. The mental static that typically accompanied her workday had diminished, replaced by a clarity that felt simultaneously foreign and familiar.

Her productivity reflected this change. Tasks that normally consumed an hour were completed in forty minutes. Problems that typically required multiple attempts yielded to first solutions. She wasn't working faster in the conventional sense—rushing or cutting corners—but with greater efficiency, her cognitive resources fully engaged rather than fragmented across multiple channels.

The revelation expanded beyond her immediate work: Had she been operating at a fraction of her potential capacity all this time, simply because her energy was being continuously siphoned away through unnoticed leaks?

The implications were both liberating and sobering. What she had previously attributed to personal limitations—moments of mental fog, difficulty concentrating, creative blocks—might have been symptoms of a fragmented attention system rather than inherent deficiencies.

She had always believed burnout resulted primarily from excessive work demands. Now she recognized a parallel truth: It also stemmed from the cumulative impact of constant interruption, distraction, and cognitive depletion—even during periods conventionally labeled as "rest."

Hour 12: Energy Without Burnout

The transformation became most apparent as Rachel left Vertex that evening. Typically, she departed the office with a familiar exhaustion—a mental depletion that left her capable of little more than basic functioning for the remainder of the day. The commute home usually passed in a blur of podcast-induced numbing or mindless scrolling, an attempt to distract herself from her own fatigue.

Tonight felt markedly different.

As she gathered her things, she realized she wasn't experiencing the usual end-of-day cognitive collapse. Her thoughts remained clear. The compulsion to immediately check her phone had diminished significantly. Most noticeably, she felt genuinely present in her body and surroundings rather than operating on autopilot.

This new state accompanied her home, where Ethan greeted her with his typical enthusiasm about a new dinosaur fact he'd learned at school. Instead of the divided attention she typically offered—one part engaged with him, another part still mentally processing work, a third part craving the distraction of her device—she found herself fully available to the conversation.

His response to this subtle shift was immediate. Rather than quickly losing interest as he often did when sensing her partial presence, he elaborated on his story, eyes bright with the rare gift of his mother's complete attention.

Rachel realized with a pang of recognition that she had been physically present but mentally elsewhere far more often than she'd acknowledged—even during moments she had specifically protected for her son.

"I've been running on empty for so long," she thought as she helped Ethan with his homework later that evening, "I had forgotten what being fully present even feels like."

The difference wasn't just about having more energy—though that was certainly true. It was about experiencing a quality of engagement that had become increasingly rare in her technology-mediated existence.

She wasn't merely reclaiming time—she was reclaiming something far more fundamental: her capacity for undivided presence.

The Big Realization: Energy Isn't Just About Work—It's About Where You Focus

After Ethan went to bed, Rachel sat in the quiet of her apartment, the day's experiment still reverberating through her awareness. Something profound had shifted in her understanding of energy management.

For years, she had approached burnout primarily as a time management problem—too many commitments squeezed into too few hours. Her recovery efforts had focused accordingly: reducing work hours, setting boundaries, and creating space in her calendar.

Yet today's experience entirely revealed a different dimension: Energy depletion wasn't just about the quantity of activity but the quality of attention she brought to each moment.

She had spent years meticulously managing external stressors without addressing the internal patterns that fragmented her focus. She had created boundaries around her time while leaving her attention completely unprotected. She had assumed that energy replenishment came primarily from rest periods, overlooking how her engagement with technology systematically prevented genuine restoration even during designated "downtime."

The insight crystallized as she sat in the stillness of her living room: She wasn't merely recovering from burnout—she was redesigning her entire relationship with attention in a world engineered to capture and monetize it.

And the first step in this transformation wasn't adding something new to her life but eliminating the systems that had been covertly extracting her most precious resource.

Rebuilding Energy in a World That Steals It

The following morning, Rachel woke with clarity beyond her immediate experiment. She was beginning to recognize how incomplete her understanding of burnout had been.

The conventional narrative she had accepted framed exhaustion primarily as the result of overwork—too many hours, too much effort, too little rest. Accordingly, the solution seemed straightforward: work less, rest more, and create better boundaries.

But her experience revealed a more complex reality.

Burnout wasn't simply about quantitative imbalances in her schedule. It represented a qualitative deterioration of her relationship with attention itself—a state where her cognitive resources were being continuously depleted not just during work hours but throughout every waking moment.

Even during periods conventionally labeled as "rest," her brain had rarely experienced genuine recovery. Instead, it had shifted from work-related processing to equally depleting patterns of fragmented attention—social media scrolling, news consumption, and entertainment designed to capture rather than restore mental energy.

The recognition was simultaneously disturbing and empowering: She couldn't address burnout simply by changing her work patterns—she had to transform her entire relationship with the technologies and systems that had commodified her attention.

Genuine recovery wouldn't come just from "resting more" but from fundamentally changing how she engaged with a world designed to extract maximum attention with minimum awareness.

The Experiment Expands: Redesigning Her Energy System

The insights from Rachel's initial 24-hour experiment demanded expansion. What had begun as a limited test revealed principles requiring broader application.

Seated at her kitchen table, the following weekend, notebook open before her, she began mapping a more comprehensive approach. This wouldn't be merely another self-improvement project, but a fundamental redesign of how she managed her most essential resource.

"I'm not actually exhausted," she wrote, the realization still striking her with its clarity. "I'm overstimulated. My energy isn't gone—it's being systematically drained through hundreds of small leaks throughout each day."

The implications extended far beyond a single day's experiment. She had been unwittingly feeding attention-capture systems that provided just enough intermittent reward to mask their cumulative cost.

Her strategy needed to match this reality in scope and ambition. One week of deliberate practice—restructuring not just how she worked, but how she engaged with the entire information ecosystem surrounding her.

She wasn't merely trying to escape burnout temporarily—she was creating conditions where burnout became structurally impossible rather than merely temporarily avoided.

Step 1: Eliminating the Hidden Energy Leaks

Rachel began with a systematic inventory, identifying every pattern, technology, and interaction that consistently depleted her energy without providing proportional value.

The list grew longer than she had anticipated, filling several pages of her notebook. The drains clustered into distinct categories, each representing a different mechanism of energy depletion:

1. The Shallow Work Trap

The constant background hum of workplace communication systems—emails requiring acknowledgment but not deep thought, slack messages interrupting focus for minimal benefit, meetings that could have been accomplished through asynchronous means.

Most insidiously, the multitasking patterns she had developed in response—rapidly switching between tasks in a way that felt productive but actually depleted cognitive resources at an accelerated rate.

2. The Decision Fatigue Drain

The countless small choices consumed mental bandwidth throughout each day—what to eat for each meal, what to wear each morning, which tasks to prioritize, when to schedule various activities.

These individual decisions seemed trivial in isolation, but collectively they depleted the same limited resource that powered creative thinking, emotional regulation, and impulse control.

3. The Information Overload Cycle
The seemingly harmless habit of "catching up" on news, scrolling through social feeds, or browsing without specific purpose. These activities created an illusion of productivity or connection while actually fragmenting attention and providing minimal lasting value.

Her brain had been trained to crave this constant input—mistaking information consumption for genuine learning or connection.

4. The Background Stress Loop
The mental bandwidth consumed by unresolved tasks, uncompleted projects, and unprocessed information—all occupying space in her working memory without active progress.

Adding to this were the emotional burdens she habitually absorbed from others—taking on colleagues' stress, friends' problems, and general anxiety from the cultural environment without conscious choice or clear boundaries.

The inventory revealed a profound truth: She wasn't exhausted merely from doing too much. She was depleted from engaging with everything in a way that systematically fragmented her attention without her awareness or consent.

With the energy leaks identified, she could now address them methodically.

Step 2: Automate, Eliminate, or Contain

Rachel established a clear framework for addressing each identified energy drain. Every item on her list would be subjected to a simple decision tree:

Automate it. Eliminate it. Contain it.

This structure transformed overwhelming awareness into actionable strategy. Each category required a different approach:

1. **The Shallow Work Trap: Contain It**
   - ☑ Emails would be processed in two dedicated sessions daily—morning and afternoon—never continuously monitored throughout the day.
   - ☑ Slack and other messaging platforms would operate with notifications disabled, accessed only during specific periods rather than allowing constant interruption.
   - ☑ Meetings would face stricter scrutiny—accepted only when her presence genuinely added value, declined when her contribution could be made asynchronously.

2. **The Decision Fatigue Drain: Automate It**
   - ☑ Breakfast became standardized—the same nutritious option each morning, eliminating one daily decision.
   - ☑ Her wardrobe was simplified into a functional "uniform" approach—coordinated options that required minimal deliberation.
   - ☑ Task prioritization would happen at the end of each day for the following day—eliminating the need to decide workflow while simultaneously trying to execute it.

3. **The Information Overload Cycle: Eliminate It**
   - ☑ Social media apps were removed from her phone, converting instant-access habit triggers into deliberate decisions requiring additional steps.

- ☑ News consumption was structured into a single daily session rather than continuous updates throughout the day.
- ☑ Random browsing during work hours was blocked through website-limiting software, creating technical barriers to unconscious habits.

4. **The Background Stress Loop: Close Open Loops**
- ☑ Unfinished tasks were captured in a trusted system and explicitly scheduled—freeing mental bandwidth previously occupied by the need to remember them.
- ☑ Emotional boundaries were established around whose stress she would absorb—recognizing that empathy didn't require taking on others' emotional states.

Rachel wasn't merely adjusting habits or implementing productivity techniques. She was fundamentally reengineering her relationship with attention itself—designing a life that protected rather than exploited her cognitive resources.

The First Day Without Energy Leaks

The morning of implementation arrived with both anticipation and apprehension. Rachel had prepared thoroughly, yet she recognized that theory and practice often diverged significantly when confronting deeply ingrained patterns.

She began with a deliberate morning routine—one that conspicuously excluded her typical digital immersion.

No phone checking before fully awake. No email review before breakfast. No diving into tasks without intentional preparation.

For the first time in years, she controlled how her brain initiated the day rather than immediately surrendering her attention to external demands.

The discomfort was immediate and physical—a restlessness in her body, an almost magnetic pull toward her devices, a sense that something essential was being missed. These sensations weren't merely psychological but represented genuine neurological craving for familiar stimulation patterns.

The experiment was revealing just how deeply her nervous system had adapted to constant input—and how uncomfortable the initial stages of recalibration would be.

The Urge to Let the World Back In

By mid-morning, seated at her desk with her modified work system in place, Rachel confronted the full force of attention addiction.

The technical aspects of her plan were functioning as designed. Notifications remained disabled across all platforms. Social media was inaccessible from her work devices. Email remained closed except during designated processing periods.

But her internal experience revealed just how powerful the conditioned responses had become.

Surprisingly, the urge to "just check" various information sources arose throughout the morning. Her mind generated increasingly persuasive rationalizations:

Surely there might be something important I'm missing. What if someone needs an immediate response? I could quickly scan headlines just to stay informed.

Beneath these surface thoughts lurked deeper anxieties: Fear of irrelevance. Concern about decreased responsiveness being interpreted as diminished commitment. Worry about missing social or cultural references that others would understand.

This wasn't merely breaking a habit—it was confronting an entire system of conditioning that had shaped her behavior for years.

Rachel recognized that this experiment extended beyond personal productivity enhancement. She was actively resisting powerful attention-capture systems designed by some of the most sophisticated psychological engineering in human history—technologies and platforms explicitly created to form exactly the dependencies she was now trying to break.

"I've been trained to be constantly available," she acknowledged silently. "Now I'm retraining my mind to protect itself."

The First Signs of Real Energy

By early afternoon, Rachel noticed a subtle but significant shift. The initial withdrawal symptoms hadn't disappeared completely, but they had diminished enough for a different quality of experience to emerge. After years of fragmented attention, her focus had developed a depth and sustainability that felt almost foreign. Complex problems that normally required multiple attempts yielded to more direct solutions—ideas connected with greater fluidity. Perhaps most notably, she completed tasks with a strange sense of completion—a satisfaction that had become increasingly rare in her reactive work patterns.

"Have I been exhausting myself all these years simply because I was never fully present?" she wondered, the question both disturbing and liberating.

The transformation extended beyond individual tasks to her overall experience of work. Without the constant neurological stimulation of notifications, alerts, and task-switching, she maintained a steadier energy level throughout the day. The usual mid-afternoon crash—typically addressed with caffeine and willpower—didn't materialize with its customary intensity.

By the time she left Vertex that evening, the experiment had yielded its most significant evidence yet:

She didn't experience the cognitive collapse that typically accompanied the end of her workday. She maintained mental presence during her commute rather than seeking distraction from her own exhaustion. Most significantly, she arrived home with energy remaining for genuine engagement with Ethan and her personal life.

The implications were profound: She wasn't operating with a fixed energy supply that work inevitably depleted. Rather, her energy had been systematically fragmented throughout each day—scattered across dozens of platforms, hundreds of micro-decisions, and innumerable distractions.

For the first time in recent memory, she was operating with her cognitive resources consolidated rather than dispersed—and the difference was transformative.

The Realization That Changed Everything

That evening, after Ethan was asleep, Rachel sat in contemplative silence, integrating the day's experiences into a broader understanding.

She had approached burnout recovery primarily through external adjustments—changing work hours, setting boundaries, and creating space in her calendar. These changes were necessary but incomplete.

What today revealed was the internal dimension of energy management—how her patterns of attention and focus determined her experience as much as her external circumstances.

She had spent years diligently defending her time from excessive demands. She had become increasingly skilled at saying no, setting limits, and creating boundaries around her schedule.

Yet throughout this process, she had left completely unprotected what was perhaps her most valuable resource: the quality and direction of her attention. She had guarded her calendar while leaving her focus vulnerable to constant exploitation.

The insight crystallized with remarkable clarity: This wasn't merely about avoiding burnout, as traditionally understood. It was about constructing an entirely different relationship with energy, attention, and presence—one that maintained vitality rather than merely managed depletion.

She wasn't just recovering from past patterns—she was designing future ones that would make burnout structurally impossible rather than temporarily avoided.

Testing the System: Can She Keep Her Energy Protected?

Rachel had dedicated a full week to implementing her new energy management system. The initial results exceeded her expectations:

Enhanced focus during work hours, reduced decision fatigue throughout the day, greater mental presence during personal time, and improved overall energy levels without increasing rest periods.

But the real challenge lay ahead: Could these changes withstand contact with a world explicitly designed to capture attention and fragment focus?

Burnout culture doesn't simply disappear because one individual chooses different patterns. Digital distraction architectures don't cease their operation because a single user implements new boundaries. Social expectations don't immediately adjust to accommodate personal transformation.

The coming days would reveal whether her newly established patterns represented sustainable change or merely temporary deviation—whether she could maintain her reclaimed energy in an environment engineered to disperse it.

The test would come not from dramatic challenges but from the subtle, persistent pressure to return to previous patterns—the accumulated weight of environmental cues, social expectations, and habitual responses that had shaped her behavior for years.

The First Attack: Digital Temptation

The initial challenge arrived through an unexpected channel. Rachel had successfully eliminated social media from her phone, removing the apps that had previously consumed hours of fragmented attention throughout each week.

The technical barrier was functioning as designed—accessing these platforms now required deliberate action rather than unconscious habit.

But systems designed to capture attention don't surrender their targets easily.

📩 **A text message from Emily vibrated her phone:** 💬 *"Did you see that viral post about the marketing industry going around? Everyone's talking about it."*

The seemingly innocent message triggered an immediate neurological response—curiosity, mild FOMO (fear of missing out), and the familiar dopamine anticipation that accompanied potential novel information.

Rachel felt the physical sensation of her attention being pulled toward the implied content—a reflexive response that bypassed conscious decision-making.

Her hands nearly moved of their own accord, ready to reinstall the app "just this once" to view the content in question.

The justifications arose automatically: *What if this contains information relevant to my work? What if I'm missing something everyone else knows about? What if this one exception is actually important?*

She recognized these thoughts not as rational considerations but as the voice of dependency—her brain's conditioned response to potential reward cues, seeking the familiar neurochemical pattern it had come to expect.

With deliberate intention, she placed her phone screen-down on the table.

If it genuinely matters, I'll hear about it through other channels.

This small moment represented a significant victory—choosing conscious engagement over reflexive response, deliberately directing her attention rather than having it captured without consent.

The Second Attack: Social Pressure at Work

The workplace presented more complex challenges to Rachel's new boundaries. While digital distraction operated primarily through technological design, professional environments added the dimension of social expectations and implicit norms.

Her new practice of checking emails only twice daily—morning and afternoon—rather than remaining in constant reactive mode had immediately improved her productivity and focus. Tasks requiring deep attention were completed more efficiently. Creative problems yielded to sustained thought.

But organizational cultures don't change to accommodate individual boundaries without resistance.

📩 **A Slack message appeared during her designated focus period:** 💬 *"Rachel, can you address this client question ASAP?"*

📩 **Shortly after, an email from her supervisor:** 💬 *"Haven't seen your response to my earlier message. Let me know your thoughts soon."*

The social pressure contained in these communications was both subtle and powerful. The requests themselves weren't unreasonable in isolation, but they represented the persistent expectation of immediate availability—the unspoken assumption that everyone should remain perpetually responsive regardless of their current priorities.

Rachel felt the familiar weight of conflicting obligations: maintaining her boundaries while also being perceived as a responsive team member.

The internal dialogue was immediate: *Am I being difficult or selfish? Will they think I don't care about my responsibilities? Should I make an exception just this once?*

But she recognized the danger in that final thought—exceptions quickly become patterns, and boundaries that bend too easily eventually break entirely.

She allowed the messages to wait until her scheduled communication period.

When she finally reviewed them hours later, she discovered what experience had suggested would be true: Neither situation had required immediate intervention. Both had resolved through other channels or simply weren't as time-sensitive as the language had implied.

This validation reinforced a critical insight: Much of what presents itself as urgent in modern work environments is merely habitual urgency—a culture of immediacy disconnected from genuine necessity.

She had won this battle not through active resistance but through the power of non-response—allowing artificial urgency to reveal itself as such through the simple passage of time.

The Third Attack: Emotional Energy Theft

While Rachel had made significant progress protecting her attention from external distractions and her time from unnecessary demands, a more subtle form of energy depletion remained to be addressed: emotional energy theft.

Throughout her life, she had unconsciously adopted the role of emotional caretaker in many relationships—absorbing others' stress, serving as a sounding board for complaints, and taking on responsibility for others' emotional states without clear boundaries.

This pattern had depleted her in ways less visible but equally consequential as work overload or digital distraction.

The test of her new boundaries arrived via text one evening:

A message from a friend:

"I really need to vent. Everything is going wrong today. Can we talk?"

Rachel felt the immediate weight of this request—the implicit expectation that she would drop whatever she was doing to provide emotional support, regardless of her own capacity in that moment.

Her conditioned response activated instantly: *I should be there for my friend. It would be selfish to say no. Their needs are more important than my boundaries.*

But her recent insights had revealed a crucial distinction: Supporting others didn't require abandoning her own well-being. Compassion didn't demand emotional absorption.

She recognized the two paths before her:

1. Absorb the emotional state, engage with the negativity, and end up depleted.

2. Offer support with clear boundaries that protect her own energy.

She composed a response that honored both her friend's needs and her own limitations:

> 💬 *"I hear you. That sounds really difficult Do you need advice on something specific, or do you just need someone to listen for a bit?"*

This simple question served multiple purposes: It acknowledged her friend's struggle, offered genuine support, but also defined the parameters of engagement rather than providing an unlimited emotional resource.

Her friend's response was revealing:

> 💬 *"I just needed to vent. Thanks for checking in. Actually writing it out already helped."*

The exchange confirmed what Rachel had suspected: Often, people don't require others to absorb their emotional state—they simply need acknowledgment and connection. By clarifying the nature of support needed, she had maintained compassion without unnecessary depletion.

This represented perhaps the most subtle victory—learning that genuine support and connection didn't require sacrificing her own emotional equilibrium.

The Moment She Knew She Was Free

As evening settled over the city, Rachel sat on her balcony reflecting on the day's challenges. She had faced three significant tests of her new energy management system:

Digital temptation pulling at her attention. Workplace expectations pressing against her boundaries. Emotional demands testing her capacity for compassionate limits.

In each case, she had maintained her new patterns—not through rigid resistance but through conscious choice about where her energy would flow.

This wasn't about selfish isolation or disconnection from responsibilities. She remained engaged with her work, responsive to genuine needs, and present for meaningful connection.

The difference lay in who controlled the flow of her attention and energy—herself or the external systems designed to capture and direct it for their own purposes.
She wasn't merely escaping burnout in its conventional sense. She was reclaiming sovereignty over her most essential resources—designing a life where she directed her energy intentionally rather than having it dispersed by default.

This realization contained power beyond any individual technique or boundary: She was no longer a passive participant in systems designed to exploit attention, but an active architect of her own engagement with the world.

The Realization That Changed Everything

For most of her adult life, Rachel had operated reactively—responding to external demands, expectations, and stimuli without questioning the cumulative impact of this orientation.

Reacting to workplace pressures. Reacting to technological notifications. Reacting to social expectations. Reacting to others' emotional states.

Each individual response seemed reasonable in isolation. Collectively, they had created a life where her energy was continuously directed by forces outside her conscious control—fragmented across dozens of platforms, hundreds of interruptions, and countless small surrenders of attention.

Now, something fundamental had shifted in her orientation:

She was acting with deliberate intention rather than reacting by conditioned habit.

She was choosing where her focus went rather than having it captured without consent. She was determining who had access to her energy rather than making it universally available.

She was structuring her engagement with time rather than being continuously pulled into urgency without distinction.

The insight clarified with remarkable simplicity: Burnout wasn't merely about working too much.

It was about losing control over where your energy flows—surrendering your most precious resource to systems designed to extract maximum value with minimum awareness.

Her recovery wasn't simply about reducing external pressures but about reclaiming internal agency—a transformation that changed everything that followed.

When Your Best Friend Doesn't Recognize You Anymore

Three weeks into her energy reclamation experiment, Rachel had established consistent new patterns:

Technological boundaries protected her attention from continuous fragmentation. Work routines that prioritized deep focus over constant reactivity. Decision systems that minimized cognitive depletion from trivial choices. Social boundaries that allowed connection without unnecessary energy absorption.

The cumulative effect had transformed her daily experience—greater clarity, sustained energy, enhanced presence, and, surprisingly, improved productivity despite less frantic activity.

But personal transformation rarely occurs in isolation. As her internal experience shifted, her external relationships began reflecting these changes—sometimes in unexpected ways.

The first significant mirror appeared in the person who knew her best.

The Rachel That Emily Knew

Emily took another sip of her coffee, studying Rachel with the combined perspective of long-time friend and trained psychologist.

"Let's start with something concrete," she suggested, setting down her mug. "When was the last time you checked your phone?"

The question landed with unexpected weight. Rachel realized she hadn't glanced at her device since arriving at the café nearly an hour earlier—a behavior that would have been unthinkable just weeks ago.

"I... don't know. Before we sat down, I guess."

A knowing smile spread across Emily's face. "Exactly. That's weird for you. Historically weird."

The observation was accurate without being judgmental. Throughout their friendship, Rachel had been the perpetually connected one—the friend who maintained constant digital awareness even during supposedly social moments.

Emily leaned forward slightly, elbows on the table. "I'm serious, Rach. You're different.

You're... present. Like, actually here. It's kind of freaking me out, to be honest."

The comment carried a lightness that softened its implications, but the underlying observation was profound: Rachel's stress patterns had become so thoroughly integrated into her identity that their absence was disorienting even to someone who cared deeply about her well-being.

She hadn't realized how completely burnout behaviors had been normalized in her relationships—how her partial presence had become an expected feature rather than recognized as a problematic absence.

The Cost of Being 'Always On'

Rachel stirred her cooling coffee, considering how to respond to Emily's observation. The realization that her former patterns had been visible to others—perhaps even more visible than they had been to herself—settled uncomfortably.

"I didn't realize how bad it was," she admitted finally, meeting her friend's gaze.

Emily's expression softened with a combination of relief and vindication. "I did."

The simple statement wasn't accusatory but reflected years of witnessing Rachel's gradual immersion in hyperconnected stress patterns. As a mental health professional, Emily had recognized the symptoms long before Rachel acknowledged them herself.

"I could always tell when you were 'here but not here,'" Emily continued, gesturing between them. "You'd be physically present, but that little crease between your eyebrows would appear, or your eyes would get that slightly unfocused look, and I knew your mind had gone back to work even if your body was still in the chair."

Rachel felt a tightness in her chest as she recognized the accuracy of this description. She had believed her divided attention was successfully concealed—that she was managing to balance social presence with professional vigilance. The illusion of this balance now collapsed under Emily's gentle but precise observation.

Emily sighed, leaning back slightly. "I just figured that's how things were. You were busy. We all are. Life in the modern world, right?"

She gestured vaguely toward the other café patrons, many of whom were engaged with devices rather than companions.

"But seeing you like this now?" Emily continued, studying Rachel with renewed attention. "It makes me wonder if we've all just been lying to ourselves about what's normal or necessary."

The observation expanded beyond their individual friendship to a broader cultural question—how collectively normalized patterns of fragmented attention and perpetual availability had reframed diminished presence as an inevitable condition rather than a problematic choice.

Rachel wasn't merely changing her personal habits; her transformation was implicitly challenging assumptions that many around her had accepted without examination.

The New Rachel—And Whether It Will Last

Rachel exhaled slowly, confronting the uncomfortable truth in Emily's observations. The person she had been—perpetually distracted, constantly monitoring digital channels, never fully present—wasn't a version of herself she wanted to reclaim.

"I don't want to be that person anymore," she said simply.

Emily nodded, genuine warmth replacing clinical observation in her expression.

"Good. Because honestly? I like this version of you better."

The affirmation carried particular weight coming from someone who had known her throughout her adult life—someone who had witnessed her pre-burnout self and could recognize authentic change rather than temporary performance.

But Emily wasn't finished. She leaned forward, pointing at Rachel with gentle challenge. "Question is... are you gonna keep this up? Or is this just one of those temporary self-improvement kicks that last until the next work crisis?"

The question addressed the central challenge of any significant behavior change:

sustainability under pressure. Many transformations appeared convincing in controlled conditions only to collapse when tested by real-world stressors.

Rachel recognized the legitimacy of this concern. She had attempted various wellness practices in the past—meditation routines that lasted a week, exercise regimens abandoned after a month, digital detoxes that ended with the first perceived emergency.

The question wasn't whether she could maintain these changes in ideal conditions, but whether they would withstand inevitable pressure to revert to previous patterns—whether her transformation represented fundamental rewiring or merely temporary deviation.

This was the real test facing her now: proving to herself and others that this reclamation of energy and attention represented permanent evolution rather than another transient self-improvement project.

The Conversation That Changed Everything

Rachel sat with Emily's question, considering its implications. She had invested significant effort in restructuring her relationship with technology, attention, and energy—but would these changes persist when challenged by old environments and expectations?

She had been so focused on establishing new patterns that she hadn't fully considered how others might perceive these changes—how her transformation might disrupt established dynamics even in her most supportive relationships.

"I'm not going back," she said finally, the statement emerging with quiet certainty rather than defensive insistence.

Emily studied her friend's expression, searching for the conviction behind the words.

Whatever she found seemed to satisfy her, a genuine smile spreading across her face.

"Good. Because I missed you."

The simple statement contained layers of meaning—acknowledgment that something essential had been absent in their connection, recognition of its return, and affirmation of its value.

Rachel hadn't fully realized how much her burnout patterns had cost herself and those who cared about her—how her fragmented presence had diminished connections even when she believed she was successfully balancing priorities.

The insight expanded her understanding of what recovery truly entailed: not merely reclaiming her own wellbeing but restoring the full potential of relationships that stress had silently eroded.

The Final Thought: Energy Isn't Just Personal—It's Relational

As Rachel walked home from the café, Emily's observations continued resonating through her awareness. She had conceptualized burnout primarily as a personal condition—her own exhaustion, her own depletion, her own compromised wellbeing.

But this framing had missed something essential: Burnout wasn't merely an individual experience but a relational one, affecting her internal state and every connection in her life.

Her stress patterns hadn't merely stolen her energy—they had systematically compromised her capacity for genuine presence with those she valued most.

Her fragmented attention had made her physically present but mentally elsewhere in countless moments with Ethan. Her perpetual work vigilance had diminished the quality of friendships, even when she made time for them. Her constant digital connection had eroded her capacity for uninterrupted engagement in all relationships.

She was recovering not just personal resources but relational ones—rebuilding her capacity for the undivided presence that meaningful connection requires.

This recognition transformed her understanding of what was at stake in maintaining her new patterns. She wasn't merely protecting her own well-being but actively reclaiming the quality of every relationship in her life.

The insight carried both responsibility and promise: Her energy management wasn't simply a personal wellness project but a fundamental restructuring of how she showed up in the world and for those who mattered most.

What Comes Next? When Stress Destroys Your Closest Connections

As twilight settled over the city, Rachel arrived home to a quiet apartment. Ethan was spending the weekend with his father, giving her rare solitude to process the day's insights.

Settling onto her couch, she found herself examining her phone with new awareness—not reaching for it habitually, but contemplating what it represented in her broader relationship patterns.

The screen displayed notifications she had once considered essential interruptions: missed calls from her ex-husband, Michael, about logistics for Ethan's school project, text messages from her boyfriend, Nathan, expressing concern about her recent unavailability, and photos of Ethan's latest dinosaur drawings that she had glanced at but never fully appreciated.

A pattern emerged with uncomfortable clarity:

> 💬 *I haven't just been absent from my friendships. I've been missing from all my relationships.*

The realization expanded beyond her conversation with Emily to encompass every significant connection in her life. Stress hadn't just depleted her personal energy—it had systematically eroded her capacity for meaningful engagement with everyone she cared about.

Her co-parenting relationship with Michael had become transactional rather than collaborative. Her romantic connection with Nathan had been squeezed into whatever time and attention remained after work demands were met. Even her relationship with Ethan—which she had tried hardest to protect—had been compromised by her divided presence during supposedly dedicated time.

As she set her phone aside without checking the notifications, Rachel recognized that her next challenge would extend beyond personal energy management to relationship repair—rebuilding connections that stress had damaged through her chronic partial presence.

This work would likely prove the most challenging phase of her recovery—acknowledging the relational cost of her burnout patterns and reclaiming not just her energy but her capacity for genuine connection with those who mattered most.

Tomorrow would bring new opportunities for presence or distraction, connection or fragmentation. For the first time in years, she felt genuinely capable of choosing the former—not because external pressures had disappeared, but because she had reclaimed the internal resources necessary to engage with them differently.

Her energy was finally her own again. Now she could decide, with clear intention, where and how it would flow.

CHAPTER 5: THE RELATIONSHIP KILLER

*The Love You Lost to Cortisol—
How Stress Destroys Relationships
Before It Destroys You*

Some Ghosts Never Leave

It takes nine months to create a relationship.

Nine seconds to destroy one.

The afternoon light filtered through Rachel's living room window, casting golden patterns across the floor where Ethan sat cross-legged, his small hands gripping colorful Lego pieces with fierce concentration. His tongue poked slightly from the corner of his mouth as he assembled his spaceship, a gesture of focus that Rachel had almost forgotten in the years she'd spent half-present in moments like these.

Just months ago, she would have missed this entirely—her body in the room but her mind buried in emails, lost in deadlines, drowning in the false urgency of work that never loved her back. She would have been seated on the couch with her laptop open, nodding occasionally at Ethan's excited commentary while her attention remained tethered to Vertex Media's endless demands.

But the memory of what had nearly happened still haunted her like a persistent shadow.

The day Ethan had stopped looking up when she entered a room.

She remembered it with painful clarity—walking into the kitchen after a particularly grueling day, expecting his usual enthusiastic greeting. Instead, he had continued coloring, his small shoulders hunched slightly, not bothering to look up. It wasn't anger or rebellion. It was something far worse: adaptation. He had simply adjusted to her emotional absence, learning not to expect connection where it had been consistently withheld.

That moment had cut through her like nothing else—not the migraines, exhaustion, or warnings from Dr. Hughes or Emily. In her son's quiet resignation, she had first truly recognized what stress was stealing from her life. Not just energy. Not just health. But the one thing more valuable than all of it—genuine connection with the people she loved.

Since that day, she had fought to repair that relationship with deliberate intention—day by day, moment by moment—slowly rebuilding trust her chronic absence had eroded. The progress was evident in small but significant ways—Ethan now seeking her out to share discoveries, his unguarded laughter when they played together, and most precious of all, the way he'd begun looking into her eyes again when she spoke to him.

Now, sensing her attention, Ethan glanced up from his creation, offering a smile that reached his eyes. "Look, Mom—it has special engines that can go to Jupiter," he explained, demonstrating how a particular piece rotated. "That's the farthest planet I want to visit."

"It's amazing," Rachel responded, genuinely present in her appreciation as she moved from the couch to the floor beside him. "Tell me more about these special engines."

The connection between them was healing—gradually, imperfectly, but genuinely.

But some relationships couldn't be saved.

Tonight, she would sit across from Nathan at dinner, facing the consequences of years of emotional unavailability in her romantic life. The thought settled in her chest with leaden certainty—some damage might be irreparable, some connections broken beyond restoration.

She watched Ethan continue building, his small hands creating something new from scattered pieces, and wondered if the same possibility existed for what remained of her relationship with Nathan.

Why High-Achievers Struggle in Relationships

Rachel initially believed burnout was neatly contained within professional boundaries—a workplace condition that could be left at the office door. However, the reality had proven far more pervasive.

Her friendships had gradually faded, contact becoming sporadic and superficial.

Her romantic relationship with Nathan now hung by fraying threads, growing more distant despite living together.

Her connection with Ethan had been rescued, but the recovery remained fragile, requiring consistent attention.

Stress hadn't merely depleted her energy—it had systematically rendered her emotionally unavailable across every meaningful relationship in her life.

🔬 Dr. Hughes explained this pattern during one of their sessions, and his expression reflected compassionate understanding rather than judgment.

"High performers don't just experience professional burnout—they experience relationship burnout," he had noted, sketching a simple diagram in his notebook. "What makes this particularly dangerous is its progression."

He had drawn three lines representing the deterioration pattern:

"It happens slowly—so gradually that you attribute changing relationship dynamics to natural evolution rather than neglect."

"It happens silently—without dramatic fights or conflicts that might alert you to the damage being done."

"And by the time you notice the full extent of disconnection, it's often too late to reverse completely."

Rachel recognized herself in this progression with uncomfortable clarity. The same traits that had made her "successful" at Vertex—her ability to prioritize work above personal needs, to remain perpetually available to professional demands, to push through exhaustion—had systematically undermined her capacity for genuine presence in her personal life.

The qualities celebrated in her professional persona had become liabilities in her most important relationships.

The Science of Stress-Induced Disconnection

🔬 During a particularly important session, Dr. Hughes had explained the neurobiological mechanisms behind Rachel's relational difficulties. The science transformed her understanding of what had happened between her and the people she loved.

> "Stress doesn't merely affect your energy levels," he had explained, sketching a diagram of neural pathways. "It fundamentally rewires your brain's capacity to connect meaningfully with others."

She had assumed her relationship challenges stemmed from simple time constraints—too many professional obligations leaving insufficient hours for personal connections. The reality proved far more complex and insidious.

> **1. Cortisol Kills Empathy**
> When chronically elevated, cortisol—the primary stress hormone—does more than prepare the body for emergencies. It actively dulls emotional sensitivity as a protective mechanism.
>
> "Your brain isn't being malicious," Dr. Hughes had explained. "It's being efficient. Under threat conditions, which chronic stress mimics, the brain prioritizes survival functions over social connection. The prefrontal cortex—responsible for empathy, nuanced emotional processing, and perspective-taking—becomes less active as resources shift toward more immediate concerns."

The result was painfully predictable: Rachel had grown increasingly distant, irritable, or emotionally shut down in personal interactions without consciously choosing or even recognizing these responses.

> **2. Dopamine Hijacks Attention**
> The neurochemistry driving high achievement often directly conflicts with what sustains intimate relationships.

> "High performers," Dr. Hughes noted, "develop dependency on the dopamine rewards that come from progress, achievement, and momentum. The brain becomes conditioned to seek these reliable chemical rewards."
>
> By contrast, meaningful relationships require qualities that don't trigger these same reward pathways: stillness, presence, patience, and comfort with uncertainty.

The resulting conflict created a pattern where Rachel grew bored, distracted, or restless during exactly the kinds of deep conversations and unstructured time that relationships need to thrive.

> **3. Adrenal Exhaustion Makes You Withdraw**
> Perhaps most damaging was the final stage of burnout, where the body's stress response system begins to falter under chronic activation.
>
> "When adrenal fatigue sets in, your nervous system initiates protective shutdown," Dr. Hughes had explained. "The brain begins interpreting all non-essential activities—including social interactions—as threatening additional demands on already depleted resources."
>
> This created a cruel paradox: Rachel began avoiding the very connections that might have supported her recovery—not because she didn't care, but because her depleted system couldn't bear the perceived energy cost of emotional engagement.

Rachel had spent years allowing this neurobiological cascade to systematically dismantle her relationships. With Ethan, she had recognized the damage in time to implement meaningful intervention. With Nathan? That remained to be seen.

Rachel's Wake-Up Call: A Conversation She Couldn't Ignore

Six months earlier, Emily had been the first to directly confront the growing distance in their friendship. The memory remained vivid—a conversation Rachel couldn't dismiss or rationalize away as she had with so many previous concerns.

They had been sitting at Reverence, their favorite coffee shop since graduate school, late afternoon sunlight streaming through windows that overlooked the park. The familiar environment only highlighted how unfamiliar their interaction had become.

Emily stirred her latte slowly, eyes fixed on the swirling pattern rather than meeting Rachel's gaze.

"I feel like I don't even know you anymore," she said finally, her voice quiet but steady.

Rachel had frowned, immediate defensiveness rising. "What? Em, we literally just had dinner last week."

Emily sighed, finally looking up. "Yeah. And the whole time, you were on your phone, answering emails, checking notifications. You asked me to repeat myself three times because you weren't listening. You were physically there, but you weren't actually there."

The observation landed with unexpected force, leaving Rachel momentarily without response. Because Emily was right, and they both knew it.

Rachel had stopped fully showing up for real moments of connection.

She had grown accustomed to being physically present while remaining emotionally and mentally elsewhere.

She had unconsciously trained her brain to prioritize digital interruptions over human connection.

"I've watched this happening for years," Emily continued when Rachel remained silent. "At first, I thought it was temporary—a busy period at work. Then I thought maybe you were just evolving different priorities. But Rachel," her voice softened with concern, "this isn't about changing priorities. You're disappearing, even when you're sitting right across from me."

That conversation had provided the first significant crack in Rachel's denial. She had recognized what was happening with Ethan and fought to repair it. But until now, she hadn't fully confronted what might be happening with Nathan.
Tonight's dinner would reveal whether that relationship could still be saved.

The Hidden Cost of Emotional Unavailability

Rachel wasn't alone in her pattern of stress-induced disconnection. Dr. Hughes had shared research demonstrating how prevalent the problem had become, particularly among high-achieving professionals.

> "Studies from relationship researchers at Gottman Institute show that chronic stress measurably reduces the brain's capacity for emotional depth," he had explained during one of their sessions. "This isn't a character flaw or a choice—it's a neurobiological adaptation with predictable relational consequences."

Three patterns emerged consistently among high achievers struggling with burnout:

1. Emotional Numbness
The brain begins suppressing deep emotional reactions as a coping mechanism for overwhelming stress. Initially, this dampens negative emotions like anxiety or frustration, but inevitably extends to positive emotions as well.

"People stop feeling excitement or sadness with their previous intensity," Dr. Hughes had explained. "They describe experiences as being 'muted' or 'distant'—almost as though they're observing their emotions rather than experiencing them directly."

This numbness creates a profound sense of disconnection from others and oneself.

2. Avoidant Communication
As mental and emotional resources deplete, conversation itself begins feeling like an unreasonable demand.

"The brain starts categorizing communication as 'high-cost,'" Dr. Hughes noted. "This leads to patterns where people keep interactions superficial to conserve energy. They unconsciously develop habits of changing subjects when conversations grow emotional, delaying responses to messages, or providing minimal engagement."

These individuals become labeled as "bad texters," "bad listeners," or "emotionally unavailable"—not because they don't care, but because their systems are conserving resources.

3. Intimacy Resistance
Perhaps most damaging in romantic relationships is how burnout affects physical and emotional intimacy.

"Romantic relationships require vulnerability, presence, and attunement," Dr. Hughes had explained. "All three demand significant energy from systems that stress has already depleted."

The predictable result: less physical attection, decreased patience during conflicts, and diminished emotional engagement—creating patterns that partners experience as rejection or indifference.

In short: Stress doesn't merely kill energy—it systematically dismantles the neurological foundations of connection.

Rachel's Realization: What Stress Had Stolen from Her Family

As Rachel's awareness expanded, so did her recognition of relationships already damaged or lost.

Her ex-husband Michael's words from their divorce three years earlier now carried new significance: "You're married to your job, Rachel. There's no room for an actual marriage alongside it." At the time, she had dismissed his complaint as unfair, even self-serving. Now, she recognized the painful accuracy in his assessment.

Ethan had gradually stopped asking her to attend school events or sports games—not because his desire for her presence had diminished, but because he had adapted to chronic disappointment. Only her recent efforts had begun rebuilding his expectation that she would actually show up.

Nathan had started seeing her less frequently over the past several months, suggesting they spend weekends apart and no longer plan the future adventures they once discussed. She initially attributed this to his busy veterinary practice but now recognized he wasn't pulling away—he was simply adjusting to the emotional distance she had already created.

One evening after beginning her recovery, while Nathan worked a late shift, Rachel found herself scrolling through old messages and photos on her phone. The evidence of her gradual disappearance from meaningful connection accumulated with each swipe:

Unanswered texts from friends who eventually stopped reaching out.

Calendar reminders for personal celebrations and milestones she had canceled for work emergencies.

Photos from Ethan's last birthday—an event she had physically attended but barely remembered, having spent most of it handling a client crisis from the hallway outside the party room.

"Oh my god," she had whispered to the empty apartment, the weight of recognition settling heavily in her chest.

She had constructed a life where work received her full attention—her complete focus, her quick responses, her best energy. Meanwhile, the people who loved her received whatever depleted fragments remained afterward.

She had initiated meaningful changes, particularly in her relationship with Ethan. But the question looming over tonight's dinner with Nathan was whether she had recognized the damage too late.

Can You Fix What Burnout Broke?

Rachel had always prided herself on her capacity to solve problems, repair what was broken, and find solutions where others saw only obstacles.

She believed her intense work ethic provided Ethan financial security after the divorce.

She had convinced herself that saying yes to every professional demand demonstrated her reliability and value.

She had assumed friends and loved ones would understand her temporary unavailability until she reached some mythical future state where balance might finally be possible.

But her recent clarity had revealed the fundamental flaws in these assumptions. She hadn't been holding everything together—she had been holding herself apart.

From the people who genuinely needed her presence, not just her productivity.

From relationships that once brought her authentic joy rather than achievement-based satisfaction.

From the version of herself capable of being emotionally present, connected, and fully alive in moments that couldn't be measured by professional metrics.

The damage was undeniable. And now, facing dinner with Nathan, the question wasn't theoretical but immediate: could genuine repair still be possible?

Consistent effort had yielded promising progress with Ethan. Their relationship was healing through daily moments of authentic connection. But romantic partnerships operated by different rules—

they required mutual investment that might no longer be available if Nathan had already emotionally withdrawn too far.

As Rachel prepared for dinner, applying minimal makeup in the bathroom mirror, her reflection revealed hope and apprehension. Some wounds could be healed with time and attention, but others left permanent scars that changed the relationship's fundamental nature. Tonight would reveal which reality she and Nathan faced.

How Stress Changes the Way We Love

Dr. Hughes had explained that burnout doesn't merely exhaust the body—it fundamentally alters how people engage in relationships, particularly intimate ones.

> "When stress becomes your default operating system," he had noted during one particularly illuminating session, "love itself begins feeling like another obligation rather than a source of replenishment."

The transformation occurs through predictable phases:

1. You Start Seeing Relationships as "To-Do List Items"

Rachel recognized this pattern immediately. Conversations with Nathan had gradually shifted from sources of connection to items requiring completion. She would find herself mentally tracking how long they had been talking, calculating when she could reasonably end the interaction to return to work tasks.

Expressions of physical affection—a hug, a hand on his shoulder, a kiss goodbye—had become automatic gestures performed without genuine presence, similar to how she would absentmindedly pet a cat while focused elsewhere.

Most tellingly, she had stopped truly listening during conversations—instead, waiting for her turn to respond or mentally addressing other concerns while maintaining the appearance of attention.

2. You Prioritize Efficiency Over Emotional Depth

As her stress levels increased, her communication patterns changed in subtle but significant ways.

She began offering quick, practical answers rather than thoughtful responses acknowledging emotional nuance.

Decision-making shifted toward pragmatic considerations rather than accounting for feelings or relationship impact.

Perhaps most damaging, she had gradually abandoned the deep, open-ended questions that explore another person's inner world, replacing them with efficient small talk that could be navigated while mentally elsewhere.

3. You Emotionally Under-Respond

The most insidious change was how stress had dampened her emotional responsiveness to others' needs and feelings.

When Nathan shared difficulties from his day, she would acknowledge them without genuine engagement—offering a distracted "That sounds hard" while continuing whatever task occupied her attention.

When friends confided in her about their struggles, she immediately offered practical advice rather than emotional validation, unconsciously treating their feelings as problems to solve rather than experiences to share.

When Ethan showed excitement about new discoveries, she would offer perfunctory appreciation—"Cool, buddy"—while her attention remained fixed on her phone or laptop.

This pattern created the most damaging aspect of relationship burnout—connection dies not through dramatic conflict but through the slow, steady erosion of emotional presence.

Rachel had exhibited every warning sign. And now, preparing to meet Nathan, she confronted the accumulated impact of years spent emotionally unavailable to the person who had loved her most consistently.

Step 1: Learning to Be Fully Present Again

Rachel had recognized she needed to begin somewhere concrete—to practice the muscle of presence she had allowed to atrophy through years of divided attention.

The first deliberate test had come with Ethan several months earlier.

On a Tuesday evening after work, Rachel had done something different rather than maintaining her usual position on the couch with laptop open while he played nearby. She had closed her computer, silenced her phone, and sat down beside him on the carpet where colorful blocks were scattered.

"Tell me about this spaceship," she had said, genuinely curious rather than performing interest.

Ethan had looked up, momentary surprise flickering across his face at this deviation from their normal pattern. He had grown accustomed to her half-presence—physically in the room but attention elsewhere.

For several heartbeats, he had studied her cautiously, perhaps assessing whether this attention was genuine or momentary. Then, hesitantly at first, he had begun explaining his creation, small hands gesturing with increasing animation as he described each component's purpose.

Rachel had made no attempt to multitask. She hadn't glanced at her phone. She hadn't mentally reviewed work tasks while maintaining eye contact. She had simply been there—fully, completely present in the moment with her son.

And something unexpected had happened: For the first time in longer than she could remember, her mind had quieted. The constant background hum of notifications, deadlines, and obligations had faded, replaced by genuine absorption in Ethan's world.

She wasn't thinking about emails waiting for response. She wasn't mentally drafting presentations or reviewing client feedback. She wasn't counting minutes until she could reasonably return to work.

She was simply present—and that presence itself had become a form of rest rather than another obligation.

This had marked the beginning of healing with Ethan—a consistent practice of full attention rather than divided awareness.

Now, as she prepared to meet Nathan, the question remained whether she could bring the same quality of presence to a relationship that might already have sustained too much damage.

Step 2: Rebuilding Friendships— One Honest Conversation at a Time

Rachel had recognized that her friendship with Emily required more than passive improvement—it needed active repair through uncomfortable honesty.

In the years of her deepening burnout, she had been an increasingly absent friend to someone who had remained consistently supportive. The patterns were undeniable:

She had canceled plans repeatedly, often at the last minute for work "emergencies."

When they did meet, she had been chronically distracted—checking her phone, mentally elsewhere, half-listening to conversations.

She had taken Emily's patience and understanding for granted, assuming the friendship could withstand unlimited neglect without consequence.

Recognition alone wouldn't heal this damage. So Rachel took an uncomfortable but necessary step: scheduling coffee specifically to acknowledge the harm and take responsibility without excuses.

When they had met at their usual café, Rachel hadn't attempted to sugarcoat her behavior or minimize its impact.

"I haven't been a good friend, Em," she had said directly, meeting her friend's eyes. "I know I've been distant and distracted for years, and I hate that I made you feel like you didn't matter. There's no justification for it—I just want you to know that I see it now, and I'm sorry."

Emily had studied her for a long moment, stirring her coffee slowly. In her silence, Rachel felt the weight of years of gradual disconnection.

"I missed you, Rach," Emily had finally responded, voice soft but direct. "But honestly? I stopped expecting you to actually show up. I adjusted to having half of your attention at best. I got used to plans being tentative based on whatever work emergency might arise."

The assessment had hurt, though Rachel recognized its complete accuracy. She had trained Emily not to expect her full presence—just as she had unconsciously trained Ethan and Nathan to adapt to her chronic emotional absence.

Rachel had swallowed hard against the tightness in her throat. "I'm here now," she had said simply. "And I don't want to disappear again. I can't promise I'll never make mistakes, but I can promise that I see what happened and I'm committed to changing it."

Emily's expression had softened slightly, a cautious smile forming. "Good. Then let's start over—no scorekeeping, just moving forward."

That conversation had been the foundation for gradually rebuilding what had been damaged. Rachel was learning that fixing relationships wasn't about grand gestures or perfect performance, but about consistent presence and honest engagement over time.

Emily had offered another chance. Ethan was responding to her renewed attention with increasing trust. But as Rachel approached the restaurant where Nathan waited, uncertainty clouded her optimism. Some relationships might have already passed the point where repair remained possible.

Step 3: Facing the Hardest Relationship of All

Rachel couldn't avoid the reality that her relationship with Nathan had suffered the most comprehensive damage from her years of emotional unavailability.

Unlike her son, who depended on her presence regardless of its quality, or Emily, whose friendship had deep roots predating her burnout, Nathan had chosen to love her—and could just as freely choose to stop.

The signs of deterioration had accumulated gradually but unmistakably. Nathan had been extraordinarily patient throughout their three-year relationship:

He never criticized her for working late or bringing projects home on weekends.

He rarely complained when date nights were canceled for work emergencies or abbreviated by early-morning meetings.

He never issued ultimatums about her availability or attention, even as both diminished.

But patience, however generous, has limits. Rachel had felt the subtle shifts indicating his withdrawal: conversations growing shorter and more superficial, physical affection becoming less frequent, and most telling, his decreasing efforts to share meaningful aspects of his life.

Love rarely ends in dramatic confrontations. More often, it fades gradually as emotional connection diminishes, leaving two people sharing space but not experience—physically together but emotionally separate.

As Rachel entered the restaurant, she spotted Nathan seated by the window at their usual table. Her chest tightened with the recognition that tonight might reveal whether enough connection remained to rebuild, or whether her awakening had come too late for this particular relationship.

The Reality of Repairing What's Broken

 Dr. Hughes had warned Rachel that fixing relationships after burnout followed different rules than personal recovery with unique challenges and limitations she needed to understand.

> "Repairing relationship damage isn't instantaneous," he had explained carefully. "It's a process that depends not just on your changes but on the other person's capacity to reinvest after being hurt."

Three principles governed the potential success of relationship repair:

1. People Don't Trust Words—They Trust Patterns

Rachel couldn't simply promise to be more present and expect immediate restoration of trust. Words alone carried little weight compared to the established patterns others had experienced.

> Real change requires consistent behavioral shifts maintained over time—a new pattern reliable enough to gradually replace the memory of previous disappointments.

2. Some Relationships Can Be Saved—Some Can't

The uncomfortable reality was that not everyone waits indefinitely for connection to be restored. Some relationships possess greater resilience to periods of emotional distance, while others reach tipping points beyond which recovery becomes impossible.

> The determining factor often isn't the severity of disconnection but its duration and the other person's individual capacity for rebuilding trust after it's been broken.

3. The Hardest Part: Accepting That You Might Have to Start Over

Perhaps most challenging was the possibility that some relationships couldn't be repaired in their current form—that genuine healing might require releasing what was and building something entirely new, or accepting that certain connections had reached their natural conclusion.

Rachel had to face this reality without allowing potential loss to drive her back toward the stress addiction that had created the damage initially. If her relationship with Nathan couldn't be saved, that loss needed to become a lesson rather than a trigger for relapse.

Recovery wasn't merely about restoring her own well-being—it required acknowledging and addressing the impact of her choices on others, whether or not those relationships could ultimately be salvaged.

As she sat across from Nathan, noting the careful politeness in his greeting that had replaced the warmth of genuine connection, Rachel recognized the extent of work required to rebuild what stress had systematically dismantled.

What If Some Relationships Don't Survive?
In the weeks preceding this dinner, Rachel had consistently worked to repair the damage stress had caused in her relationships.

She was showing up reliably for Ethan, being genuinely present for homework, attentive to his stories, and attending school events with her full attention rather than divided focus.

She was making time for Emily, their friendship gradually regaining its former depth through consistent engagement and honest communication.

She was learning to be present in all interactions, practicing the skill of undivided attention that burnout had eroded.

Yet despite these genuine improvements, one relationship continued feeling increasingly distant. Nathan remained kind, patient, and supportive—but something essential had changed. The warmth that had characterized their early connection had faded to polite affection. Conversations that once flowed naturally now felt carefully navigated. The quiet comfort of genuine intimacy had been replaced by the careful choreography of people sharing space but not inner worlds.

The most unsettling realization was that these changes persisted despite her efforts to reconnect— suggesting that the damage might have crossed a threshold beyond which repair wasn't possible.

Because sometimes, even after genuine change, people don't wait. They adapt, they protect themselves, they move forward in ways that no longer include the connection that once existed.

The Psychological Cost of Slowing Down

Dr. Hughes had explained that stepping away from stress addiction creates unexpected challenges beyond the neurochemical withdrawal—particularly in confronting the full impact of one's absence on important relationships.

> "Many people focus so intensely on their own recovery that they're unprepared for the relational consequences that become visible only after the fog of burnout begins clearing," he had noted during a particularly difficult session.

Rachel was experiencing this reality directly as her improving awareness revealed the extent of disconnection stress had created in her personal life.

Three psychological patterns made this recognition particularly challenging:

1. The "Relationship Debt" Effect

Just as Rachel had accumulated cortisol debt through years of chronic stress, she had simultaneously built relationship debt with those she loved—a deficit of trust, intimacy, and connection created through consistent emotional unavailability.

> Like financial debt, this relational deficit couldn't be eliminated through a single payment or grand gesture. It required consistent investment over time, with no guarantee that the relationship could be fully restored to its previous condition.

2. The "Too Little, Too Late" Syndrome

For some relationships, there exists a point beyond which the damage becomes functionally irreversible—not because repair is theoretically impossible, but because the injured party has already completed their emotional processing of the loss.

> When someone has already grieved a relationship while technically still in it, they may have little motivation to reinvest in rebuilding connection, having already adapted to its absence.

3. The Identity Shift Complication

Perhaps most challenging was the reality that Rachel wasn't merely changing her schedule or communication patterns—she was fundamentally transforming who she was and how she engaged with others.

The people in her life had built relationships with the workaholic, stress-addicted version of Rachel—adapting their expectations and behaviors to accommodate her limitations.

Now they faced the complex task of deciding whether they wanted to build a relationship with this emerging version of her—a process requiring reassessment rather than simple continuation.

Rachel was confronting the uncomfortable truth that recovery wasn't just about personal transformation—it included accepting that some relationships might not survive the very changes necessary for her well-being.

The Science of Relationship Damage from Chronic Stress

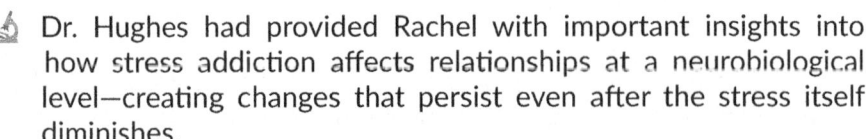 Dr. Hughes had provided Rachel with important insights into how stress addiction affects relationships at a neurobiological level—creating changes that persist even after the stress itself diminishes.

> "Chronic stress doesn't just strain relationships temporarily," he had explained. "It creates neurological adaptations in both parties that fundamentally alter how connection functions."

Three primary mechanisms create lasting relationship damage:

1. Long-Term Stress Triggers Emotional Disengagement
When consistently exposed to a partner's emotional unavailability, the brain eventually learns to disconnect as a protective adaptation—reducing expectations for engagement to avoid repeated disappointment.

This neurological adjustment doesn't immediately reverse when the stressed individual becomes more available. Even when stress symptoms subside, the emotional dampening often persists as a protective mechanism.

The result: Partners stop expecting emotional intimacy, cease initiating vulnerable conversations, and no longer express needs they've learned won't be met—creating a relationship pattern of mutual withholding that becomes self-perpetuating.

2. Dopamine-Rewired Priorities
The stress-addicted brain develops dependency on the dopamine rewards that come from work challenges, deadlines, and crisis management. By comparison, relationships begin feeling unsatisfyingly slow, unpredictable, and lacking in measurable outcomes.

High achievers unconsciously prioritize professional contexts where feedback is immediate and accomplishment clearly defined over relationship investments where progress remains intangible and metrics nonexistent.

The result: The brain forms increasingly strong associations between progress/satisfaction and work environments, while relationships become categorized as maintenance activities rather than sources of fulfillment.

3. Unintentional Neglect Creates Emotional Scar Tissue
Perhaps most damaging is how chronic emotional absence literally reshapes relationship expectations at a neurological level.

Initially, a partner experiences pain when connection is consistently unavailable. Over time, however, the brain adapts by reducing the importance of that connection—literally rewiring neural pathways to depend less on a relationship that proves unreliable.

This adaptation doesn't immediately reverse when the formerly absent partner becomes available again. The protective neural patterns remain, creating what functionally resembles emotional scar tissue—areas where vulnerability once existed but has been covered by protective barriers.

The result: Even when a burnout sufferer genuinely changes and becomes emotionally available, their partner may have already completed the neurological adaptation of learning not to need them—a change not easily reversed through simple reassurance or renewed attention.

Rachel recognized with growing concern that Nathan might have already undergone this adaptation—not from lack of care, but as a natural protective response to years of her emotional unavailability.

Rachel's Breaking Point: The Dinner That Said Everything

Rachel had been genuinely trying to rebuild the connection with Nathan over the past several weeks.

She had initiated more meaningful conversations beyond daily logistics.

She had become religious about putting her phone away during their time together. She had created space for genuine connection without work interruptions.

But something felt fundamentally different—as though she was the only one still fighting for the relationship. Nathan remained unfailingly kind, but his responses had grown shorter, his questions less probing, his overall engagement polite rather than passionate.

Seated across from him at Emilio's, their favorite Italian restaurant, the distance between them felt more significant than the physical table separating them. The candlelight cast soft shadows across his familiar features as he responded to her questions about his day with well-constructed but emotionally neutral answers.

Politeness—that was what troubled her most. The careful pleasantness that replaces genuine connection when relationships begin fading. Not anger, not conflict, but something far more concerning: indifference disguised as courtesy.

Rachel felt her chest tighten with recognition. She set down her fork beside her barely-touched risotto and met his eyes directly.
"Are we okay?" she asked, her voice steady despite the apprehension beneath it.

Nathan looked up, momentary surprise crossing his features at the directness of the question. Something flickered in his expression—a brief vulnerability quickly contained.

He didn't answer immediately. That hesitation alone confirmed what she had feared—the pause containing all the uncertainty their relationship had become.

Finally, he sighed, shoulders releasing tension he'd been carrying throughout the meal.

"I don't know, Rach," he admitted, voice gentle but honest.

The three words landed with the weight of finality. Not because they offered certainty, but because they acknowledged the uncertainty that had grown between them—the space where connection had once existed, now filled with careful distance.

That was the moment she truly recognized that despite her recent changes, she might have already lost him—not to another person or dramatic conflict, but to the slow erosion of trust that occurs when someone learns they cannot depend on your presence.

The Hard Truth: Some Relationships Don't Heal

Rachel had focused so intently on her personal recovery that she hadn't fully confronted an uncomfortable possibility: What if some connections were already damaged beyond repair?

Not because Nathan didn't care for her—his kindness and patience demonstrated otherwise. Not because she didn't genuinely want to rebuild their relationship. But because the version of Rachel he had fallen in love with hadn't been consistently present for years, and the emotional adjustments he had made in response couldn't be easily reversed.

🔬 Dr. Hughes had prepared her for this possibility, though the reality proved more painful than theoretical discussions had suggested.

> "Three factors determine whether a relationship can recover from burnout-induced damage," he had explained during a session that now felt prophetic.

1. Recovery Takes Time—But Some People Move On First

The neurological and emotional adaptations created in response to chronic disconnection don't instantly reverse when one partner begins changing. While healing remains theoretically possible, it requires both parties' active investment in rebuilding.

If one person has already completed their emotional processing of the relationship's decline—grieving its loss while technically still participating in it—they may lack motivation to reinvest in its restoration.

2. Some Damage Can't Be Undone

Consistent emotional unavailability creates specific patterns of hurt that persist beyond behavior change. Being repeatedly deprioritized establishes deep trust issues regarding one's importance in another's life.

Even after genuine transformation, some partners struggle to believe the change will last—having adapted to disappointment as the relationship's defining pattern rather than its exception.

3. Guilt Doesn't Fix What's Broken

Rachel experienced profound guilt about her years of emotional neglect—the missed opportunities for connection, the half-presence she had offered, the consistent prioritization of work over relationship.

But guilt itself provides no foundation for rebuilding a genuine connection. Relationships recover through consistent presence and rebuilt trust, not through remorse about past failures.

"Guilt can actually become counterproductive in relationship repair," Dr. Hughes had explained during one session. "It often drives performative efforts or creates pressure that makes organic reconnection more difficult."

The emotion served as important recognition of past patterns but offered little constructive energy for building new ones. No amount of retrospective regret could rewrite interactions that had already occurred.

Rachel was confronting the hardest truth of her recovery journey: changing herself didn't guarantee she could change relationship outcomes that her previous patterns had set in motion.

The Conversation She Had Been Avoiding

Rachel had always identified as a problem-solver—the person who fixed crises at work, managed challenges efficiently, and pushed through obstacles rather than surrendering to them. In her professional life, sufficient effort and skill had reliably produced desired outcomes.

But relationships operate by different rules—rules she was only now beginning to fully comprehend.

Sometimes, despite genuine care and renewed effort, timing determines outcomes more than intention.

That evening after dinner, she and Nathan sat on opposite ends of her couch, the space between them symbolic of the emotional distance that had grown. The apartment was quiet save for the distant hum of traffic outside, the silence stretching uncomfortably between them.

Rachel finally gathered her courage and asked the question she had been avoiding for weeks: "Do you still love me?" Her voice was steady despite the vulnerability the question revealed.

Nathan exhaled slowly, turning toward her. His eyes held the same gentleness they always had—the kindness that had initially drawn her to him.

"Yeah, Rach. I do," he answered quietly, his tone containing both honesty and resignation.

The confirmation should have brought relief, but instead, it made her chest tighten with recognition of the deeper problem.

"Then why does it feel like we're already over?" she asked, finally giving voice to the sensation that had been growing despite her efforts to deny it.

Nathan was quiet for a long moment, his expression thoughtful as he considered her question. When he finally spoke, his words carried the weight of realization that had been forming over months.

"Because love isn't the problem," he said finally. "It's everything else."

The simple assessment contained profound truth. Love had remained—their basic care and concern for each other still existed. What had disappeared was the connection that transformed love from concept to experience—the moment-by-moment attunement, vulnerability, and presence that constituted genuine intimacy.

Rachel understood with painful clarity: the damage was real, and despite their mutual care, love alone wasn't sufficient to repair what years of emotional distance had broken.

Learning When to Let Go

🔬 During a particularly important session, Dr. Hughes had explained that emotional recovery includes developing discernment about relationships—knowing when continued effort serves healing and when acceptance of natural endings becomes necessary.

> "Part of maturity is recognizing that not all relationships are meant to be permanent," he had noted gently. "Some serve important purposes for specific life chapters before reaching their natural conclusion."

Three principles guided this difficult discernment:

1. **If You're the Only One Trying, It's Not a Partnership—It's a Rescue Mission**

Rachel needed to honestly assess whether Nathan remained actively invested in rebuilding their connection. Relationships require mutual effort, particularly during healing phases. If one person carries the entire reconnection weight, the imbalance becomes unsustainable.

The most loving choice sometimes involves recognizing when someone has emotionally moved beyond the possibility of recommitment, regardless of how much you wish otherwise.

2. **The Past Can't Be Rewritten—Only the Future Can Be Built**

No amount of present effort could erase the accumulated impact of years spent emotionally unavailable. Rachel couldn't undo the missed opportunities for connection or the pattern of deprioritization Nathan had experienced.

Real healing required acknowledgment of what had been lost rather than attempts to minimize or dismiss it—building a new foundation rather than trying to repair one that had been fundamentally compromised.

3. **Sometimes, Love Exists But The Relationship Doesn't Work Anymore**

The most painful realization was that mutual care could coexist with relationship dysfunction. Nathan's continued affection wasn't in question. The issue was whether the relationship itself could still function as a source of genuine connection and growth for both participants.

Rachel faced the difficult task of determining whether staying reflected authentic possibility or merely fear of acknowledging what had already ended.

As she sat with Nathan in the growing understanding of their situation, Rachel had no clear answers about what came next—only the growing recognition that some decisions can't be forced through willpower alone.

The irony wasn't lost on her: She had begun repairing her relationship with Ethan just in time to save their bond. However, with Nathan, time appeared to be running out, regardless of her genuine desire for a different outcome.

When Love Isn't Enough

Days after their conversation, Rachel sat in her car outside Vertex Media, gripping the steering wheel so tightly her knuckles whitened. She had done everything she knew to do—made herself consistently available, prioritized their time together, demonstrated through actions rather than just words that she had genuinely changed.

And yet, it still wasn't enough.

The realization challenged her fundamental beliefs about how life worked. She had always operated according to a straightforward equation: sufficient effort plus correct strategy would inevitably produce desired outcomes. This principle had proven reliable throughout her professional life—consistent effort generally yielded proportional results.

But relationships don't operate by these mechanical rules. They function as complex systems requiring mutual investment, appropriate timing, and sometimes, an element beyond rational control—the mysterious chemistry that either remains or dissipates based on factors no amount of intentional effort can fully address.

She was confronting the uncomfortable truth that relationships aren't projects to be managed through efficient execution. They don't respond reliably to effort alone. They require two people who remain genuinely invested in meeting at a point of authentic connection.

And for the first time in their relationship, Rachel wasn't certain that Nathan still occupied that meeting point, regardless of how much she wished otherwise.

The Psychology of Relationship Drift

🔬 During a particularly insightful session, Dr. Hughes explained how stress addiction creates specific patterns of relational deterioration that persist even after stress levels normalize.

> "Chronic stress doesn't just temporarily strain relationships," he had noted. "It fundamentally alters relationship dynamics in ways that create persistent patterns even after the original stress triggers diminish."

Four specific mechanisms create what relationship researchers call "emotional drift"—the gradual separation of partners despite continued physical proximity:

1. The High-Performer Guilt Loop

Rachel recognized this pattern immediately. Her awareness of having been emotionally absent generated intense guilt, which then drove compensatory perfectionism in her attempts to reconnect.

Rather than allowing natural, imperfect reengagement, guilt pushed her toward performative effort—trying too hard, monitoring responses too closely, creating subtle pressure that made organic reconnection more difficult.

The resulting dynamic created a self-reinforcing cycle where guilt drove effort, but the effort itself felt forced rather than natural—further complicating authentic connection.

2. Burnout Warps the Way You See Your Partner

When operating under chronic stress, the brain begins categorizing all non-work activities—including relationships—as either obligations or interruptions rather than sources of replenishment.

Over time, this categorization becomes internalized. Expressions of affection begin registering as demands rather than invitations, and requests for attention feel like additional burdens rather than opportunities for connection.

The more stress dominates, the more one unconsciously withdraws from authentic engagement—creating a pattern that doesn't automatically reverse when stress levels change.

3. Emotional Absence Becomes the New Normal

Partners initially notice and react to emotional unavailability. They express needs, request attention, and actively seek reconnection.

After sufficient time without response, however, they adapt. They stop expecting presence, cease initiating vulnerable conversations, and develop independence from the emotional resources previously sought in the relationship.

This adaptation serves as psychological protection—and once established, it doesn't immediately disappear when the unavailable partner becomes available again.

4. Reconnection Feels Foreign, Even After Burnout Ends

When Rachel finally began making herself genuinely available, Nathan had already adapted to her chronic absence—not through resentment but through necessary emotional self-protection.

He had learned not to depend on her presence, not to expect her full attention, not to need the connection that had proven unreliable. These adaptations weren't conscious choices but psychological adjustments that had become his new normal.

This explained the quiet tragedy of relationship burnout: The damage often becomes functionally permanent, not in dramatic moments of conflict, but in the gradual adaptation that occurs while both people remain physically present but emotionally separated.

Rachel was now facing this reality directly—the possibility that Nathan's emotional adaptations to her absence had become so thoroughly integrated that reconnection might no longer be possible.

The Talk She Wasn't Ready For

A week after their initial conversation, Rachel and Nathan sat facing each other in her living room, the weight of unresolved questions hanging between them. Early evening light filtered through the windows, casting long shadows across the hardwood floor.

This was the discussion they had both been postponing—the one that would determine whether they continued together or acknowledged what seemed increasingly inevitable.

Rachel gathered her courage, forcing herself to ask the question directly.

"Do you think we can fix this?" Her voice remained steady despite the vulnerability the question revealed.

Nathan rubbed his temples slightly before meeting her gaze, his expression reflecting genuine care and unmistakable resignation.

"I don't know, Rach," he answered after a moment, the honesty in his voice more telling than the words themselves.

She hated that answer, primarily because she recognized its meaning beneath the surface:

uncertainty. "I don't know" rarely meant genuine indecision in these contexts; it typically signified a conclusion already reached but difficult to articulate.

She exhaled sharply, feeling emotion tightening her throat.

"I love you, Nathan. I don't want to lose this," she said, the words emerging with unexpected intensity.

He sighed, his expression softening with genuine affection despite the distance between them.

"I love you too," he replied, the words sincere despite what followed. "But this isn't just about love."

There it was—the truth she had been resisting fully acknowledging. Their problem wasn't the absence of care or affection. The issue lay in the connection itself—the day-to-day experience of genuine presence and intimacy that formed the foundation of sustainable partnership.

Love remained, but the relationship infrastructure that translated that love into lived experience had been systematically compromised over years of emotional distance.

And sometimes, love alone isn't sufficient to rebuild what extended neglect has damaged.

The Three Hardest Truths About Relationship Burnout

🔬 Dr. Hughes had provided Rachel with several difficult but necessary insights about relationships damaged by chronic stress—principles that were proving painfully relevant to her situation with Nathan.

1. People Move On Emotionally Before They Move On Physically
The presence of someone in a relationship doesn't necessarily indicate their continued emotional investment. Partners often complete their grieving process while still physically present—continuing to participate in relationship routines while having internally accepted its effective conclusion.

By the time direct conversations about relationship status occur, one person has typically processed much of their emotional response to the disconnection, creating an imbalance where one partner begins the separation conversation while the other only begins processing it.

2. Trust in Emotional Availability Is Hard to Rebuild
People develop lasting psychological responses to repeated experiences of emotional neglect or deprioritization. These patterns create specific neural pathways that don't immediately restructure when circumstances change.

Even after genuine transformation, the memory of emotional unreliability persists—creating hesitation before reinvesting vulnerability in a connection that previously proved inconsistent.

3. Love Alone Doesn't Heal Wounds—Consistency Does
Dramatic gestures, intense conversations, or passionate reconnections provide poor foundations for relationship repair. Genuine healing requires the steady accumulation of reliable presence over time.

People instinctively trust patterns over promises, consistent behavior over intermittent intensity. If the essential connection hasn't been reconstructed through patient, consistent engagement, affection alone cannot sustain the relationship.

Rachel was recognizing the painful application of these principles to her situation with Nathan. While she had been awakening to the importance of their connection, he had been gradually adapting to its absence—learning to function independently of the emotional resources their relationship had once provided.

Even as she successfully rebuilt her bond with Ethan through patient, consistent attention, she watched her relationship with Nathan move toward what increasingly appeared to be its natural conclusion.

The Moment She Had to Let Go

Rachel felt tears forming despite her effort to maintain composure, her voice slightly unsteady as she asked the question they had both been avoiding.

"So... is this it?" The words hung in the air between them, finally giving voice to what had been developing for months.

Nathan didn't answer immediately. The pause itself communicated more than words could have—the silence contained acknowledgment rather than uncertainty.

Finally, he exhaled slowly, meeting her gaze with genuine sadness and resolution. "I think we've been over for a while," he said quietly. "We just didn't want to say it."

The words landed with finality despite their gentle delivery. The weight of recognition settled fully upon her—not as sudden revelation but as confirmation of what she had been gradually understanding despite her resistance.

Rachel nodded slowly, tears falling freely now but without the intensity of fresh grief. This was acknowledgment rather than revelation—naming what had already happened rather than creating something new.

There were no raised voices, no accusations, no dramatic gestures. Just two people who had once created a genuine connection finally acknowledged its completion—the natural conclusion to a process that had been happening beneath their conscious awareness for longer than either wanted to admit.

That was perhaps the hardest aspect to accept: Their relationship hadn't ended in dramatic conflict or betrayal, but through the quiet erosion of connection that occurs when presence is consistently withheld, regardless of intention.

The Aftermath: Learning to Live Without What She Lost

The days following their conversation passed in a peculiar emotional fog for Rachel. She moved through necessary routines—work responsibilities, household tasks, and coordinating Ethan's schedule with Michael—while processing the reality of Nathan's absence from her future.

Her body had gradually adjusted to operating without chronic stress chemicals, but now she faced adapting to life without someone who had been emotionally significant for years. The silence of her apartment felt heavier during evenings after Ethan returned to his father's house, previously familiar spaces now containing the conspicuous absence of Nathan's presence.

The particular pain wasn't in losing someone suddenly, but in recognizing they had been incrementally disappearing long before physical separation occurred. The relationship had been fading gradually, with subtle adjustments and accommodations masking the growing distance until it could no longer be ignored.

She sat alone on her couch one evening, staring at nothing in particular, when her phone vibrated with an incoming message.

📩 Emily: "Hey. I know you're hurting. Let me come over?"

Rachel hesitated briefly. Her previous pattern during emotional difficulty had been isolation—withdrawing to process privately while projecting competence and control to others.

But that pattern represented the behavior that contributed to her relationship difficulties. The version of herself she was working to become approached connection differently—acknowledging vulnerability rather than disguising it, inviting support rather than projecting self-sufficiency.

She picked up her phone and typed a response that represented small but significant growth:

💬 *"Yeah. I'd like that."*

She had lost an important relationship, but she wasn't surrendering to the patterns that had created that loss. She would continue building meaningful connection where it remained possible—with Ethan, with Emily, with others who remained present in her life.

Tomorrow, she would pick up her son from Michael's house. Their healing relationship continued strengthening through her consistent presence and attention—tangible evidence that some connections could be restored through persistent, genuine engagement.

That growth represented the victory she would focus on—the relationship she had recognized as endangered in time to implement meaningful change.

When the Damage Hits You All at Once

Rachel had initially conceptualized burnout as a dramatic event—a sudden collapse, a definitive breaking point, a moment of unmistakable crisis. This framing had prevented her from recognizing its actual progression in her life.

The reality had proven far more insidious. Burnout hadn't arrived suddenly but had developed incrementally over years—each small compromise, boundary violation, and prioritization of work above well-being contributing to the gradual erosion of her health, energy, and relationships.

By the time she recognized the pattern, significant damage had already accumulated across multiple domains of her life. She had spent years borrowing energy from her future—living on stress hormones her body couldn't indefinitely sustain. Now, her relationships had experienced something similar—emotional bankruptcy after years of connection withdrawal.

The most painful aspect of this recognition was its uneven impact across her life. With Ethan, she had identified the damage early enough to implement meaningful intervention—watching with profound gratitude as their bond gradually strengthened through her consistent presence and attention.

With Nathan, awareness had come too late—the adaptations to her chronic emotional absence had already restructured the relationship beyond what could be repaired, regardless of her genuine desire for a different outcome.

The lesson emerged with uncomfortable clarity: Not everything damaged by stress could be restored through the same recovery process. Some losses represented permanent consequences of patterns that had operated too long without intervention.

The First Day Without Him

Rachel woke alone in her apartment, the space beside her in bed unfilled for the first week since she and Nathan had acknowledged their relationship's conclusion—the morning light filtered through partially closed blinds, illuminating a room that felt simultaneously familiar and strange.

Seven days had passed since their conversation—a week of adjusting to new routines, explaining the situation to concerned friends, and navigating the practical logistics of separating lives that had grown intertwined. She had moved through these tasks with a strange combination of grief and functionality, mourning what had been lost while handling necessary arrangements.

No strategy could erase this particular pain. No checklist could efficiently process the emotional complexity of significant relationship loss. This wasn't a challenge to be overcome through increased effort or improved technique—it was an experience to be fully acknowledged and gradually integrated.

She rose from bed, made coffee in the kitchen that suddenly felt too large for one person, and caught her reflection in the window overlooking the city. The face looking back at her showed evidence of recent difficulty but also emerging resilience.

She was still here, still functioning, still moving forward despite significant loss.

And though part of her instinctively wanted to retreat into familiar patterns—working longer hours, seeking distraction through increased responsibility, numbing emotion through productivity—she recognized these impulses as the very behaviors that had contributed to her relationship difficulties.

Today, she would pick up Ethan for their weekend together. She would be fully present with him, continuing to strengthen the connection she had nearly lost before recognizing its vulnerability. She would maintain the practices that supported her recovery rather than abandoning them during emotional challenges.

This represented the genuine test of her transformation: Could she experience authentic pain without reflexively returning to stress addiction as emotional anesthetic? Could she allow natural grief without seeking escape through workaholism or performance-based validation?

The Guilt That Comes With Healing

Rachel sat across from Emily at The Reverence, their familiar coffee shop providing comfortable context for difficult conversation. She stirred her rapidly cooling drink absentmindedly, attention focused inward rather than on the motion.

Emily watched her with the combination of professional insight and personal concern that characterized their friendship, allowing silence until Rachel seemed ready to engage.

"So this is the new you, huh? Post-Nathan?" Emily finally asked, her tone gentle despite the directness of the question.

Rachel attempted a smile that didn't quite reach her eyes. "I guess so."

Emily leaned forward slightly, elbows on the table. "How are you actually handling it? The real answer, not the polite one."

Rachel hesitated before answering, considering how to articulate the complex emotional landscape she was navigating.

"Honestly? I'm split in two," she admitted finally. "Part of me feels... lighter. Like I'm not constantly failing at something impossible. The other part feels like I'm drowning in what might have been if I'd woken up sooner."

The assessment was accurate. She did feel lighter—freed from attempting to repair what had become irreparable, released from constantly measuring the gap between Nathan's response and their former connection. But she simultaneously experienced profound sadness—mourning not just the relationship itself, but the version of herself who had believed professional achievement could substitute for genuine presence without consequence.

Emily tapped her fingers gently against her mug, considering her friend's words. "You're allowed to be sad, you know. This is a real loss."

Rachel sighed, her gaze dropping briefly. "I know. I just... I feel guilty. Like I'm only dealing with this now, after the damage has already been done. Like I should have seen it earlier, should have changed sooner."

That represented the most difficult aspect of her current emotional process—recognizing how much had been lost that might have been preserved with earlier awareness, accepting the permanent consequences of patterns she had only recently understood.

Later that afternoon, as she engaged fully with Ethan—truly present, genuinely connected during their trip to the science museum—she experienced both gratitude and grief simultaneously. Gratitude for the relationship she had managed to save through timely intervention.

Grief for what had been permanently lost despite her genuine desire for different outcome.

This represented the complex reality of stress recovery: not everything damaged could be restored, but what remained intact could still be nurtured toward health and beauty.

The Reality of Rebuilding After Relationship Burnout

Dr. Hughes had cautioned Rachel that the most challenging aspect of emotional recovery wasn't the initial recognition or even the necessary behavioral changes—it was navigating the aftermath as greater awareness revealed the full extent of what had been compromised.

> "Recovery doesn't immediately deliver relief," he had explained during a particularly important session. "It often begins with increased pain as improved awareness reveals damage that was previously obscured by stress chemicals and defense mechanisms."

Three specific challenges characterize this phase of healing:

1. You Start Seeing the Damage More Clearly

As stress chemicals diminish and defensive numbing fades, emotional sensitivity returns—often bringing heightened awareness of relationships that suffered during burnout periods.

Memory functions differently without chronic stress hormones, allowing clearer recall of missed opportunities, moments of disconnection, and patterns of unavailability that contributed to relationship deterioration.

This increased clarity often produces intense regret as the full impact of stress-driven behavior becomes undeniable—creating a painful but necessary foundation for genuine change.

2. People Don't Immediately Trust the New You

Behavioral changes, however genuine, don't immediately erase others' adaptive responses to previous patterns. Those who experienced chronic emotional unavailability develop protective mechanisms that persist beyond the behavior that triggered them.

People remember and respond to established patterns rather than recent improvements—creating frustrating situations where genuine transformation remains unrecognized or untrusted for significant periods.

This delayed recognition creates particular difficulty during recovery, as the improved behavior doesn't immediately produce improved relationships.

3. The Loneliness Hits Before the Healing Does

Perhaps most challenging is the temporary increase in emotional isolation that often accompanies early recovery. As artificial sources of validation and distraction diminish, genuine connection hasn't yet been fully rebuilt.

Rachel had broken free from toxic work patterns, but this liberation initially increased her awareness of disconnection rather than immediately replacing it with a healthy relationship.

Her relationship with Nathan had ended, removing a significant source of companionship, however compromised it had become.

Without the constant stimulation of workplace crisis or relationship management, she faced herself more directly—a necessary but initially uncomfortable experience that preceded genuine healing.

This transition period represented perhaps the greatest vulnerability for relapse into stress addiction—the temporary increase in emotional discomfort creating temptation to return to familiar patterns of numbing through overwork and performance-based validation.

Making Sure This Never Happens Again

The loss of her relationship with Nathan represented both ending and beginning—the conclusion of a significant chapter in her life and the initiation of a new approach to connection that might prevent similar patterns in future relationships.

Rachel couldn't change what had already occurred, undo the accumulated impact of years spent emotionally unavailable, or rewrite the history that had led to this particular relationship's conclusion.

But she could integrate this experience as meaningful guidance for future choices—allowing this loss to inform rather than define her ongoing development.

The story with Nathan had concluded, but numerous other relationships continued evolving. The question wasn't whether she could recover what had been lost, but whether she could create different patterns moving forward—building connections characterized by genuine presence rather than partial attention.

This journey was just beginning, with each authentic interaction representing a small but significant step toward the person she was becoming rather than the stress-addicted achiever she had been.

Final Thought: The Warning You Can't Ignore

Through painful experience, Rachel had discovered burnout's most significant relationship impact:

Stress doesn't merely damage physical health—it systematically erodes the capacity for genuine connection with others.

This erosion occurs long before it becomes visible, operating in seemingly insignificant moments that cumulatively create profound disconnection.

It happens during physically present but mentally absent interactions—when bodies occupy the same space while attention remains elsewhere.

It develops when urgent work consistently takes precedence over meaningful conversation—when deadlines repeatedly outrank relationships in priority sequencing.

It grows when professional demands consume emotional resources—leaving nothing but depletion by the time personal interactions occur.

While physical burnout symptoms could be addressed through changed behaviors and recovery practices, relationship damage followed different rules. Once chronic disconnection had persisted sufficiently long, some bonds couldn't be restored regardless of genuine desire or effort.

The most sobering reality—typically omitted from conventional burnout recovery literature—was that genuine healing didn't guarantee relationship restoration. You could transform yourself completely while still experiencing the permanent consequences of previous patterns.

As Rachel tucked Ethan into bed that evening—fully present, genuinely connected during their bedtime story routine—she experienced simultaneous emotions that might once have seemed contradictory: genuine grief over what had been irretrievably lost with Nathan alongside authentic hope about what continued developing with her son.

This represented both warning and promise: once damaged by chronic stress, relationships don't automatically heal when stress diminishes. Some connections, once broken, remain permanently altered. Others, recognized in time, can gradually strengthen through consistent attention and authentic presence.

Rachel had lost her relationship with Nathan—a genuine cost of patterns she had maintained too long without awareness or intervention. But she remained committed to ensuring no other significant connections suffered similar fate.

She would transform her relationship with presence itself—making conscious choices about attention allocation rather than unconsciously prioritizing productivity above connection.

She would continue building what could still be saved.

What Comes Next? The Hidden Bill Your Body Never Forgets to Collect

As Rachel continued navigating the aftermath of her relationship loss while strengthening remaining connections, she noticed something unexpected: Despite significant improvements in her stress management, technology boundaries, and relationship presence, she still experienced periods of profound physical depletion.

These episodes didn't correlate with current stress triggers or work demands. They seemed to arise randomly—days where her body felt unusually heavy, her thinking foggier than usual, her energy mysteriously diminished despite adequate rest and nutrition.

During a session with Dr. Hughes, she finally articulated the question that had been forming:

> "Why do I still feel physically depleted sometimes? I've changed my habits, improved my boundaries, transformed my relationship with work—but my body seems to be holding onto something I can't identify."

Dr. Hughes nodded with recognition, having anticipated this phase of her recovery.

"What you're experiencing isn't random," he explained. "You're encountering what researchers call 'allostatic load'—the accumulated physical impact of chronic stress that remains in the body long after the behaviors that created it have changed."

Rachel was beginning to understand that stress leaves more than psychological and relational consequences—it creates biological debt that the body methodically collects, often long after the original stress patterns have been addressed.

Discovering the nature of this cortisol debt—and developing strategies to address its persistent physical impact—would become her next challenge in the ongoing journey toward genuine recovery.

CHAPTER 6: THE CORTISOL DEBT

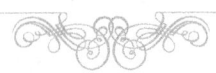

The Debt You Didn't Know You Owed—Every Stressful Day Lives in Your Body, and It's Time to Pay the Bill

The Ghost in Your Body: When Your Past Comes to Collect

Rachel woke up screaming at 3:17 AM.

Her heart hammered against her ribs as if trying to escape. Sweat soaked through her sheets, the cotton clinging uncomfortably to her skin. Her body hummed with electric panic, neurons firing warning signals with no actual threat to respond to.

But there was no crisis demanding her attention. No looming deadline threatened her career. No emergency required her immediate response.

She'd been implementing consistent stress-reduction practices for months. Her relationship with Ethan had been steadily healing through dedicated attention and genuine presence. She'd even begun finding a measure of peace in the aftermath of her relationship with Nathan ending.

Yet her body was reacting as if she were still drowning in the overwhelming demands that had characterized her previous life at Vertex Media.

As her breathing gradually slowed, her pulse reluctantly settling into a more sustainable rhythm, a terrifying question formed in her mind:

💬 *What if getting out of stress is only half the battle?*

The memory of Dr. Hughes' warning—delivered months earlier but dismissed at the time—returned with uncomfortable clarity.

💬 *"Your body keeps the score, Rachel. Every time you used stress as fuel, you weren't creating energy—you were borrowing it. And that debt compounds with interest."*

She'd successfully escaped the addiction to stress chemicals, dismantling the patterns that kept her perpetually overwhelmed. But sitting in her darkened bedroom, heart still fluttering from the phantom emergency her body had manufactured, she confronted a sobering reality:

She couldn't outrun the bill her years of stress had accumulated. The collection notice had arrived, and her body was demanding payment.

The Debt You Never Knew You Were Accumulating

Rachel had believed that implementing proper boundaries, reducing work hours, and developing healthier habits would quickly restore her to optimal functioning. The hard part, she assumed, was breaking the addiction to stress itself—after that, recovery would follow a predictable upward trajectory.

But her body wasn't adhering to the timeline her mind had established.

Despite her genuine progress in stress management, she continued experiencing unexplainable symptoms that seemed disconnected from her current lifestyle:

Random crashes of fatigue descended without warning, even after nights when she'd slept soundly for eight hours or more.

Memory gaps appeared during conversations—momentary blank spaces where familiar names or concepts should have been, followed by frustrating brain fog that made simple tasks require conscious effort.

Inexplicable body aches developed in her lower back, shoulders, and joints, accompanied by digestive issues that emerged despite no significant changes to her diet.

Most perplexing was a persistent inability to feel genuinely rested—regardless of how much sleep she got or how effectively she managed her current stress levels.

During her weekly session with Dr. Hughes, he explained the physiological reality she was facing with characteristic directness.

"Think of stress like a credit card," he said, leaning forward slightly in his chair, his expression serious but compassionate. "For years, you've been charging energy to that card. You might have stopped making new purchases, but the balance? It's still there. With interest."

The metaphor illuminated her current situation with uncomfortable clarity. Rachel hadn't merely been managing stress poorly—she had systematically accumulated a cortisol debt. And now, her body was sending the collection notice, regardless of her current improved habits.

The Science of Physiological Debt

Throughout her high-pressure career, Rachel had relied on stress to push beyond normal human limitations. When exhaustion threatened to slow her down, she hadn't rested—she had deployed stress hormones to override her body's natural signals.

What she hadn't realized was that she wasn't creating energy from nothing. Each time she pushed through fatigue with another coffee, another deadline-driven adrenaline spike, another "I'll sleep when this project is done" bargain, she was effectively taking a loan from her future self.

🔬 **Dr. Hughes explained the biology behind this process:**

> "Stress isn't energy—it's a hormonal override that forces your body to perform beyond its sustainable capacity," he explained, sketching a simple diagram showing how stress hormones affect various bodily systems. "It's like removing the governor from an engine—you get more power temporarily, but you're causing damage with every minute you operate beyond specifications."

This system worked remarkably well in the short term—which explained why so many professionals became dependent on it:

A rush of adrenaline helped her meet impossible deadlines, providing laser-like focus and suppressing basic needs like hunger or fatigue.

Cortisol spikes kept her alert during exhausting meeting marathons, creating an artificial sense of importance around every task.

Norepinephrine floods gave her that energized feeling of control during chaos, making stress oddly addictive despite its damaging effects.

The fundamental problem was that the body maintains perfect accounts of these transactions. Unlike financial debt that can be forgiven or discharged through bankruptcy, physiological debt remains on the books—and the body never forgets to collect.

How Rachel Discovered Her Cortisol Debt

Rachel had been diligently implementing all the right changes to her lifestyle:

She had established firm boundaries around work, including a strict "no emails after 8 PM" policy that she maintained without exception.

She had stopped skipping meals to complete "just one more task," prioritizing regular nutrition over manufactured urgency.

She had developed the skill of saying no to requests that would overextend her resources, protecting her time and energy with newfound determination.

By all conventional measures, she had broken her addiction to stress. She had transformed her habitual patterns. She had created sustainable practices that should have restored her vitality.

So why did she feel so depleted despite these positive changes?

One morning, leaning closer to the bathroom mirror to apply concealer, she noticed the persistent dark circles beneath her eyes. The dullness in her normally clear skin. The slight tremor in her hands as she attempted precision with her makeup brush.

These weren't merely symptoms of current stress—they represented the accumulated interest payments on years of physiological debt. She had stopped borrowing from her future, but the principal remained, silently compounding with each passing day.

And as she was discovering, no amount of green smoothies, meditation apps, or wellness routines could magically erase the biological reality of what her stress addiction had cost her.

The Three Stages of Cortisol Debt (And How to Know Where You Are)

🔬 During an extended session focused specifically on her lingering symptoms, Dr. Hughes explained that cortisol debt operates similar to financial debt—with predictable stages of accumulation and consequences.

"At first, it feels like a solution rather than a problem," he noted, his expression reflecting years of experience with burnout patients. "The extra energy seems like an advantage. But if you don't pay it off regularly through adequate rest and recovery, it compounds—and eventually, your body implements forced collection through symptoms you can't ignore."

The challenge, he explained, is that most people don't recognize they're accumulating cortisol debt until they've reached advanced stages where recovery becomes significantly more difficult.

"Understanding which stage you're in helps determine the appropriate recovery approach," he continued, opening a notebook to outline the progression.

1. Stage One: The "Overdraft" Phase (Early Warning Signs)

What Happens in This Stage?

> During this initial phase, the body begins relying on stress hormones to push through natural tiredness. Function remains generally normal, but energy levels become increasingly unstable—creating a roller-coaster effect of high performance followed by crashes.

Warning Signs:
Caffeine dependence develops, shifting from enjoyment to necessity for normal functioning.

Performance actually improves under pressure, but significant energy crashes occur when the pressure lifts.

Sleep becomes more difficult as the mind resists "turning off," despite physical tiredness.

Rachel recognized she had spent years in this stage without acknowledging the pattern, dismissing early warning signs as simply part of a high-performance career.

2. Stage Two: The "High-Interest" Phase (Chronic Fatigue Sets In)

What Happens in This Stage?

> The body begins showing unmistakable signs of hormonal overload. Energy becomes not just unstable but unpredictable—waking up exhausted despite adequate sleep becomes common. Focus and motivation become increasingly difficult to maintain without external pressure.

Warning Signs:
Morning fatigue persists regardless of sleep duration or quality.

Brain fog and forgetfulness appear in situations that previously posed no cognitive challenge.

The paradoxical state of feeling simultaneously wired and tired becomes common—restlessness combined with exhaustion.

Dr. Hughes identified this as Rachel's current position—months into her recovery but still experiencing the accumulated effects of years in cortisol debt.

3. Stage Three: The "Bankruptcy" Phase (Your Body Shuts Down)

What Happens in This Stage?

> In this advanced phase, the stress response system itself begins to fail. Stress hormones no longer provide their former boost—they simply make the person feel worse. Emotional numbness, disconnection, and physical illness become prevalent as the body implements increasingly desperate measures to force rest.

Warning Signs:
Profound exhaustion persists regardless of rest attempts.

Mood disturbances, including anxiety, depression, or emotional flatness, develop or intensify.

A sense of dissociation from oneself emerges—feeling like an observer of one's life rather than a participant.

Rachel had briefly experienced this stage during her worst burnout period—and was determined never to return to that state of physiological bankruptcy.

"The longer you remain in cortisol debt," Dr. Hughes concluded, "the higher the price you pay—and the longer the recovery period takes."

Having identified Rachel's current position in the debt cycle, the next step was determining exactly how deep her debt had grown over years of stress addiction.

Are You in Cortisol Debt? Take This Quick Test

In order to develop an appropriate recovery protocol, Dr. Hughes had Rachel complete a specialized assessment to measure her cortisol debt level.

"Before we can create a repayment plan, we need to understand the full extent of what we're dealing with," he explained, handing her a simple questionnaire. "Answer honestly—no one benefits from minimizing what's happening."

Answer YES or NO to the following:
1. Did you regularly push through exhaustion for years, assuming you'd "rest later"?
2. Do you still feel tired—even after a full night's sleep?
3. Did you rely on caffeine, adrenaline, or stress to function for extended periods?
4. Do you still feel restless when things are too calm?
5. Do you struggle to truly relax—even during vacations or downtime?
6. Do you frequently feel overwhelmed by small tasks or decisions?
7. Have you noticed memory issues, brain fog, or mood swings?
8. Do you get sick often or have unexplained physical symptoms?

Rachel answered yes to six of the eight questions, scoring well into the severe range on the assessment.

"This confirms what I suspected," Dr. Hughes noted as he reviewed her responses. "You're dealing with significant cortisol debt—even though you've broken the addiction pattern, your body is still operating in a substantial deficit."

The implications were clear: The debt was real and measurable and wouldn't simply disappear because she had stopped accumulating more. Like any significant debt, it required a deliberate, structured repayment plan—not just hope that it would somehow resolve on its own with time.

The Wake-Up Call: What Happens If You Ignore Cortisol Debt?

The assessment results helped Rachel understand why she wasn't feeling fully recovered despite her progress in stress management. The persistence of her symptoms wasn't a sign of failure in her current approach but rather evidence of how deeply the previous patterns had affected her physiology.

"I've been thinking about this all wrong," she realized during a morning when sleep disturbances had once again left her feeling depleted despite following all her new healthy habits. "I thought I just needed to stop the stress, but it's more complicated than that."

The metaphor Dr. Hughes had introduced resonated with increasing clarity:

She wasn't just tired—she was operating in a physiological deficit that had accumulated over the years.

She didn't just need rest—she needed a systematic approach to repaying the energy she had borrowed from her future self.

And if she didn't address this debt directly, her body would continue forcing collection through increasingly disruptive symptoms.

This wake-up call shifted Rachel's understanding of recovery. She couldn't simply manage stress better moving forward—she needed to actively repair the damage that had already occurred through deliberate, scientifically-informed practices designed specifically for cortisol debt repayment.

The Real Cost of Cortisol Debt — What Happens When You Ignore It?

For years, Rachel had been taking out stress loans against her body's energy reserves:

She borrowed from adrenaline when natural fatigue should have signaled time for rest.

She relied on caffeine and artificial deadline pressure to maintain productivity when her natural energy had been depleted.

She perpetually promised herself she would "rest later" when important projects were completed—yet that rest was inevitably postponed by the next urgent task.

But she had never actually repaid what she had borrowed—creating a mounting debt that her body was now determined to collect.

"Cortisol debt doesn't simply vanish when you improve your habits," Dr. Hughes had warned. "Think of it like financial debt—stopping new credit card charges is essential, but the existing balance continues accruing interest until specifically addressed."

Even with her significant lifestyle improvements, Rachel's body continued operating in a deficit state. The symptoms she experienced weren't merely lingering effects that would naturally fade with time—they were her body's increasingly insistent payment demands for years of overlooked energy loans.

The Four Ways Your Body "Collects the Payment" for Cortisol Debt

Years earlier, when Rachel had first consulted him about occasional fatigue, Dr. Hughes had warned her about the potential consequences of continued stress patterns.

> "Your body will always settle its debts," he had cautioned, his expression serious. "If you don't stop borrowing from stress and start repaying what you've already borrowed, it will force collection in ways you won't appreciate."

At the time, Rachel had nodded politely while internally dismissing the warning as overly dramatic. Now, experiencing the reality of cortisol debt collection firsthand, the accuracy of his prediction was undeniable.

The collection process typically follows a predictable pattern—beginning subtly but becoming increasingly difficult to ignore as the debt grows.

1. The Energy Crash — You Wake Up Tired No Matter How Much You Sleep

Rachel had implemented exemplary sleep hygiene—early consistent bedtime, completely dark room, no electronic devices, comfortable temperature. But despite these positive changes, she frequently woke feeling as if she hadn't rested at all.

Why This Happens:
Chronic stress fundamentally disrupts normal sleep architecture, preventing the body from properly cycling through essential deep and REM sleep phases even when sleep duration seems adequate.

Elevated evening cortisol levels keep the brain in a state of hypervigilance, maintaining a subtle "high alert" mode that prevents truly restorative rest.

Perhaps most significantly, the body literally forgets how to generate energy through normal physiological pathways, having relied too long on emergency stress hormones for basic functioning.

Symptoms Rachel Still Experienced:
Morning grogginess persisted despite sleeping 8+ hours in optimal conditions.

A profound afternoon energy crash appeared reliably around 2-3 PM, resistant to even high-quality nutrition or moderate caffeine.

She had begun relying on strategic naps simply to function through complete days—something previously unnecessary in her high-energy lifestyle.

These weren't merely signs of current fatigue but her body's insistent collection notices for years of accumulated energy debt.

2. Emotional Burnout — You Stop Feeling Joy, Excitement, or Motivation

Despite meaningful progress in rebuilding her relationship with Ethan and establishing healthier work-life boundaries, Rachel occasionally experienced periods of unexplainable emotional flatness—as if observing life through a slightly frosted window that dulled both negative and positive feelings.

Why This Happens:
Sustained stress exposure progressively desensitizes the brain's dopamine system—the neurochemical network responsible for motivation, pleasure anticipation, and reward processing.

Elevated cortisol levels directly suppress serotonin production, creating biochemical conditions that make experiencing joy and satisfaction increasingly difficult.

The brain's threat-detection systems remain hyperactivated, directing energy toward survival functions rather than positive emotional experiences—making everything feel subtly harder, less rewarding, and more effortful.

Symptoms Rachel Was Noticing:
Occasional periods of diminished interest in activities she intellectually knew she enjoyed. Episodes of emotional numbness during what should have been meaningful moments.

Times when she needed to consciously force engagement in social situations or personal interests, despite genuinely wanting to be present.

These emotional symptoms weren't character flaws or signs of depression but the neurochemical consequences of years operating under chronic stress conditions.

3. Health Crashes — Your Body Develops Symptoms Doctors Can't Explain

Rachel had begun experiencing health disruptions that didn't correlate with any clear cause:

Tension headaches developed with increasing frequency despite improved ergonomics and reduced screen time.

Digestive sensitivities appeared without corresponding dietary changes.

Her skin began reacting to products she had used for years without previous issues.

Why This Happens:
Prolonged cortisol elevation significantly suppresses immune function, creating increased vulnerability to routine infections and inflammatory conditions.

Chronic stress triggers systemic inflammation—the body's nonspecific response to perceived threats—leading to seemingly random pain patterns, digestive disturbances, and allergy-like reactions.

The autonomic nervous system remains stuck in sympathetic dominance (fight-or-flight mode), creating a constellation of physical symptoms that appear to lack an obvious medical explanation.

Symptoms Rachel Was Experiencing:
Increased frequency of minor illnesses despite maintained nutrition, hydration, and sleep practices.

Development of seemingly random physical complaints—joint discomfort, muscle tension, skin sensitivity—without clear injury or trigger.

Medical evaluations consistently returned "normal" results despite her subjective experience of distinctly abnormal physical sensations.

These physical manifestations weren't imaginary or psychosomatic; they were the body's increasingly urgent signals that previous stress patterns had created genuine physiological damage requiring specific attention.

4. The Nervous System Meltdown — You Stop Feeling Like Yourself

Perhaps most disconcerting for Rachel was an occasional sense of disconnection from herself—brief periods when she felt like a stranger in her own life, observing her activities with a peculiar sense of distance.

Why This Happens:
Extended exposure to stress hormones literally rewires neural circuitry, creating heightened baseline reactivity to potential threats while dampening response to positive stimuli.

The nervous system becomes effectively trapped in survival mode—a physiological state designed for short-term emergency response rather than ongoing function.

Over time, stress responses become so deeply integrated into identity and function that their absence creates a disorienting sense of unfamiliarity with oneself.

Symptoms Rachel Recognized:
Episodes of depersonalization feeling oddly detached from her experiences, as if observing rather than participating in her own life.

Difficulty remembering what genuine calm felt like—her "normal" had been defined by stress for so long that its absence created a strange identity vacuum.

Occasional existential uncertainty about whether she would ever feel fully "like herself" again—not recognizing that her previous "self" had been fundamentally shaped by stress chemistry.

These experiences weren't psychological disturbances but the natural consequence of a nervous system trained for continuous emergency response, attempting to adapt to non-emergency conditions.

The Emergency Cortisol Reset Protocol

After reviewing the extent of Rachel's cortisol debt symptoms, Dr. Hughes didn't minimize the challenge ahead or offer false reassurance about quick fixes.

"You've spent years accumulating this debt," he explained with compassionate directness. "You can't expect to pay it off overnight or through superficial changes. But we can start the repayment plan—right now—with specific protocols designed to address what's happening physiologically."

Rachel needed more than generic stress management techniques or wellness platitudes. She required a comprehensive cortisol reset—a systematic approach to rebuilding her body's energy reserves and rewiring her nervous system from the ground up.

> The structured plan Dr. Hughes developed contained three essential phases, each addressing a specific aspect of stress recovery:
>
> 1. **Stop adding new debt** — Eliminate all remaining sources of unnecessary cortisol elevation
> 2. **Reset the nervous system** — Restore normal function to stress response mechanisms
> 3. **Rebuild energy reserves properly** — Develop sustainable energy without stress as a crutch

This wasn't about managing stress better—it was about complete physiological rehabilitation from years of hormonal overload.

Step 1: Stop Taking Out New Stress Loans (Breaking the Debt Cycle)

Although Rachel had already implemented significant changes to reduce her overall stress levels, Dr. Hughes identified several subtle ways she continued "borrowing" from her energy reserves without recognizing these patterns as problematic.

📝 How to Stop Adding New Stress Debt Immediately:

1. The Unnecessary Urgency Detox

Most stress doesn't emerge from genuine emergencies but from responding to routine situations with emergency-level physiological reactions. Rachel needed to refine her system for evaluating what truly deserved immediate attention versus what could be approached with appropriate perspective.

Her refined protocol included:

Removing all mobile notifications except calls from Ethan—eliminating the constant stream of micro-interruptions that triggered small but cumulative cortisol spikes throughout each day.

Establishing clear, written criteria for what constitutes genuine urgency in professional contexts, requiring conscious evaluation rather than reflexive response to every request labeled "ASAP."

Developing a personal mantra, she repeated when feeling the pull of artificial urgency: "Not everything urgent is important, and not everything important is urgent."

2. The Digital Stress Loop Reset

Rachel hadn't fully appreciated how significantly her nervous system reacted to even brief digital exposures. Each time she checked her phone—even without notifications—her brain initiated a subtle threat-scanning process, elevating stress hormones in preparation for potential problems.

Her enhanced protocol addressed this pattern:

No phone exposure during the first 90 minutes after waking—allowing her body to establish natural energy rhythms before introducing potential stressors.

Complete elimination of notifications after 7 PM—creating a digital sunset aligned with her body's natural cortisol reduction timeline.

Establishment of specific "information consumption" windows rather than continuous availability—training her brain to process inputs in batches rather than remaining constantly vigilant.

3. The Caffeine Reset

Despite her improved habits, Rachel continued using caffeine as an energy supplement rather than for occasional enjoyment. Dr. Hughes helped her understand that caffeine doesn't generate energy—it forces the adrenal glands to produce stress hormones, creating artificial stimulation at the cost of deeper energy depletion.

Her modified approach included:

Strict limit of one coffee before noon—preventing afternoon consumption that would interfere with natural cortisol reduction.

No caffeine within 10 hours of bedtime—allowing complete clearance before sleep cycles begin.

Replacement of afternoon coffee with adaptogenic herbs specifically selected to support adrenal function rather than forcing additional output.

4. The Stress Tolerance Test

Rachel had significantly improved her stress response but needed greater refinement in distinguishing between productive challenge and unnecessary stress. She implemented a simple but effective self-assessment:

Any time she noticed a stress response beginning, she paused to ask: "Is this truly urgent, or am I creating an emergency where none exists?" When the answer revealed unnecessary stress activation, she immediately implemented a pattern-interruption technique to prevent cortisol elevation from continuing.

Through these focused interventions, Rachel eliminated virtually all remaining sources of unnecessary cortisol elevation—creating the essential foundation for addressing her accumulated debt.

Step 2: Reset Your Nervous System

With unnecessary stressors eliminated, Rachel needed to address the more fundamental problem—a nervous system that had been operating in high-alert mode for so long it had forgotten how to function differently.

🔬 **Dr. Hughes provided a comprehensive protocol for resetting stress response mechanisms in real time:**

"Think of this as teaching your nervous system a new language," he explained. "Right now, it only knows how to speak 'stress.' We need to help it remember that other states exist and how to access them reliably."

The three-part protocol addressed immediate stress responses, stuck activation patterns, and long-term neural rewiring.

1. 90-Second "Stress Interrupt" Technique (Stop Cortisol Spikes in Real Time)

Rachel had already developed basic skills for reducing stress reactivity, but some triggers still activated her nervous system automatically through pathways established over years of conditioning.

🔬 **Dr. Hughes enhanced her approach with a more sophisticated technique based on research showing that emotional responses typically last about 90 seconds unless reinforced:**

> **Specific Protocol:** The moment a stress response began, Rachel would:
>
> Take a deep breath, counting slowly to four during inhalation.
>
> Exhale for a longer duration than the inhale—ideally six to eight counts—sending a direct signal to the parasympathetic nervous system that danger had passed.

> Add multisensory grounding—pressing her feet deliberately into the floor, touching different textures with her fingertips, naming colors in her environment—to activate brain regions that counteract stress response.
>
> Repeat this cycle three times, approximately 90 seconds total.

This technique interrupted the cortisol cascade before it could fully develop, preventing minor triggers from escalating into extended stress states.

With consistent practice, Rachel developed near-complete control over her stress response—breaking the automatic cortisol cycle that had dominated her physiology for years.

2. The 60-Second Cold Reset
(Trick Your Nervous System into "Safe Mode")

Despite her improved regulation skills, Rachel occasionally experienced periods where her nervous system seemed stuck in high-alert mode—unable to downregulate despite cognitive recognition that no emergency existed.

 Dr. Hughes introduced a physiological intervention based on the mammalian dive reflex—a phenomenon where cold exposure to the face triggers immediate parasympathetic activation:

> **Specific Protocol:**
> Adding a 30-second cold shower at the end of each morning shower—not merely uncomfortable but genuinely cold enough to trigger the physiological response.
>
> Keeping ice packs in the freezer for rapid stress resets during the day—applied to the face, back of the neck, and wrists for 60 seconds when feeling overwhelmed.

> Splashing genuinely cold water on her face and submerging her wrists under cold water for 30-60 seconds when experiencing stress activation that wouldn't dissipate through breathing alone.

This technique utilized the body's evolutionary wiring to force a switch from sympathetic (stress) to parasympathetic (recovery) dominance almost instantly.

Rachel found this intervention particularly effective during periods of stubborn activation—her heart rate would visibly slow, breathing would deepen, and mental clarity would return within moments of cold application.

3. The 5-Minute "Brain Rewire" Exercise (Reprogram Your Cortisol Response)

Rachel's brain had spent years forming associations between productivity and stress activation—creating neural pathways that automatically initiated stress responses in work contexts regardless of actual threat levels.

🔬 Dr. Hughes provided a targeted neuroplasticity exercise designed to create alternative neural pathways:

> **Specific Protocol:**
> Find a quiet location free from distractions or interruptions.
>
> Recall a recent situation that would typically trigger stress activation—visualizing it in detail but without generating the stress response.
>
> Mentally rehearse handling the same situation with complete calm and effectiveness—creating vivid imagery of productivity paired with physiological equilibrium rather than emergency response.

> Engage all sensory systems in this visualization—what would be seen, heard, felt, even smelled and tasted when responding from a place of calm competence rather than stress activation.

This practice utilized directed neuroplasticity—the brain's ability to form new neural connections through focused attention and repetition—to create alternative response pathways that didn't require stress activation for effective function.

Through consistent implementation of this three-part protocol, Rachel's nervous system gradually established a new baseline—one where calm represented the default state rather than a temporary exception.

With her nervous system reset underway, she could finally address the third essential component of recovery: rebuilding genuine energy reserves.

Step 3: Rebuild Your Energy Without Stress (Training Your Body to Function Without Cortisol Spikes)

The final phase presented perhaps the greatest challenge. Rachel had relied on stress chemistry for energy production for so long that her body had largely forgotten how to generate and sustain energy through normal physiological pathways.

"This is where most recovery attempts fail," Dr. Hughes explained. "People eliminate obvious stressors and perhaps reset their immediate responses, but never rebuild their fundamental energy systems. Without that step, relapse becomes almost inevitable when facing significant challenges."

Rachel needed to retrain her body to produce sustainable energy without relying on emergency stress hormones as a crutch.
Replace Stress-Driven Work with Flow State

Rachel's work approach had historically relied on deadline pressure and crisis response to generate focus—a common but depleting strategy. She refined her methodology to emphasize flow state instead:

She restructured her schedule around 120-minute deep-focus sessions with complete immersion in single tasks—creating the conditions for flow state to emerge naturally rather than forcing productivity through stress.

She eliminated all potential distractions during these periods and developed a consistent pre-work ritual that signaled to her brain that focus time was beginning—creating reliable entry points to flow without requiring stress as a trigger.

The result was paradoxical but powerful: she accomplished more substantive work while experiencing less stress—replacing frantic multitasking with sustained, effective attention.

1. Use "Reverse Deadlines" to Break the Panic Habit

Rachel had unconsciously trained herself to rely on last-minute pressure for motivational fuel—creating artificial emergency where none was necessary. She reversed this pattern:

Rather than waiting for deadline pressure to motivate completion, she established personal deadlines well ahead of official requirements—removing the artificial urgency that had previously served as motivational fuel.

She built deliberate recovery periods after task completion rather than immediately launching into the next obligation—creating positive reinforcement for early completion rather than rewarding last-minute panic with relief.

This approach delinked productivity from stress, teaching her system that effectiveness didn't require emergency-level hormonal states.

2. Make Calm Feel More Rewarding Than Stress

Perhaps most fundamental was addressing the subtle reward system her brain had established around stress itself. Rachel had unconsciously learned to associate stress with productivity, meaning, and value—making calm feel empty by comparison.

She systematically rewired this association:

She began consciously celebrating moments of calm effectiveness rather than stress-fueled "heroics"—creating new positive associations with balanced energy states.

She established specific "rest rewards" following accomplishments—reinforcing that rest represented productive recovery rather than laziness or missed opportunity.

These deliberate interventions gradually shifted her internal reward system away from stress-based validation toward recognition of sustainable effectiveness.

By the end of this phase, Rachel's body had begun relearning how to generate and maintain energy through normal physiological pathways rather than constant emergency mobilization.

For the first time in years, she experienced genuine vitality rather than the artificial stimulation of stress hormones—a profound shift from merely surviving to actually thriving.

Final Warning: If You Don't Pay Off Your Cortisol Debt, Your Body Will Force You To

Rachel had waited years to address her accumulated cortisol debt, but now she was implementing a systematic repayment plan based on physiological reality rather than wishful thinking.

Most people never reach this stage of recognition and response. They continue borrowing against their future well-being until the system finally collapses completely—forcing recovery through illness, breakdown, or complete incapacitation.

The body maintains perfect accounts of stress chemistry, and the collection methods grow increasingly painful when voluntary repayment isn't initiated.

Rachel's experience demonstrated both warning and possibility: The debt accumulates silently but can be addressed through deliberate, scientifically-informed interventions before catastrophic collection becomes necessary.

The key insight remained clear: You can recover from cortisol debt—but only by acknowledging its existence and creating a structured repayment plan that addresses the physiological reality rather than merely the symptoms.

The Hidden Interest Rates of Cortisol Debt — Why It Costs More Than You Think

As Rachel implemented her comprehensive debt repayment strategy, she noticed something unexpected: Despite significant improvements in her stress management, certain symptoms persisted—evidence that cortisol debt carries consequences beyond the immediate energy depletion.

She had stopped taking out new stress loans through conscious boundary setting.

She had reset her nervous system through targeted interventions designed to restore normal function.

She had begun rebuilding her energy reserves through sustainable practices rather than emergency chemistry.

But her body continued showing subtle signs of past damage—indications that cortisol debt doesn't simply disappear once new habits are established but leaves lasting effects that require specific attention.

The longer stress debt remains unaddressed, the more extensive this collateral damage becomes—creating what amounts to "interest payments" on the original debt.

Rachel was learning through firsthand experience that stress debt doesn't merely deplete energy in the moment but creates lasting changes that can persist long after the original patterns have been modified.

The Five "Interest Fees" of Long-Term Cortisol Debt

🔬 During an extended session focused on these persistent effects, Dr. Hughes explained that full recovery requires addressing not just the energy depletion aspect of stress but the secondary damages it creates in multiple body systems.

"Think of it this way," he suggested. "Every time you borrow from stress, you pay more than just the principal amount. There's interest accruing in different aspects of your physiology—and the longer you wait to address it, the higher that interest climbs."

Rachel was experiencing five specific "interest payments" on her years of accumulated stress debt:

1. Your Metabolism Slows Down (You Gain Weight Even If You Eat the Same)

For years, Rachel had maintained relatively stable weight despite inconsistent eating patterns. Recently, however, she'd noticed changes in her body composition despite maintaining similar nutrition and exercise routines.

Why This Happens:
Cortisol directly triggers fat storage, particularly in the abdominal region—an evolutionary adaptation designed to create energy reserves during perceived famine or threat.

Prolonged stress exposure fundamentally alters metabolic function—downregulating systems to conserve energy when the body perceives ongoing threat.

Stress chemistry creates specific cravings for high-energy foods—particularly sugar, refined carbohydrates, and other rapidly available energy sources—further compromising metabolic balance.

Symptoms Rachel Was Experiencing:
Weight gain concentrated primarily around her midsection despite maintaining consistent nutrition and exercise habits.

Intensified cravings for sugary foods and simple carbohydrates, particularly during periods of fatigue.

Digestive changes, including bloating and food sensitivities, seemed disconnected from specific dietary choices.

Rachel had effectively forced her body to operate on emergency chemistry for years—and now her metabolism remained locked in protective mode, conserving resources as if still under threat.

This metabolic disruption required specific interventions beyond general stress reduction before the damage would begin to reverse.

2. Your Brain Shrinks (Memory, Focus & Mental Sharpness Decline)

Despite significant improvements in her stress management, Rachel occasionally experienced cognitive difficulties that would have been uncharacteristic for her before burnout—moments where mental clarity that once came effortlessly now required conscious effort.

Why This Happens:
Prolonged cortisol exposure literally shrinks the hippocampus—the brain region responsible for memory formation, learning, and cognitive flexibility.

Chronic stress significantly reduces cerebral blood flow, limiting the oxygen and nutrient delivery essential for optimal brain function.

Sustained emergency states keep the brain prioritizing reactive threat assessment over higher executive functions like creative problem-solving and nuanced analysis.

Symptoms Rachel Still Noticed:
Occasional word-finding difficulties during conversations—moments where familiar terms seemed temporarily inaccessible.

Brief episodes of entering rooms, forgetting her purpose, or losing her train of thought mid-sentence.

Periods of mental fog during complex tasks that previously would have engaged her full cognitive capacity without effort.

These weren't simply signs of aging or normal fluctuations in attention. They represented actual neurological changes resulting from years of stress exposure—changes that required targeted rehabilitation rather than merely stress reduction.

3. Your Sleep Gets Worse (Even When You Feel Exhausted)

Rachel had implemented exemplary sleep hygiene practices, yet continued experiencing nights where genuine restorative sleep remained elusive despite profound exhaustion.

Why This Happens:
Cortisol directly suppresses melatonin production—the hormone essential for initiating and maintaining sleep cycles—creating a biochemical barrier to restorative rest.

Chronic stress conditions the nervous system to remain partially vigilant even during sleep, preventing full entry into the deepest, most regenerative sleep phases.

Prolonged stress alters normal sleep architecture—disrupting the balance of REM and deep sleep necessary for complete recovery and cognitive processing.

Symptoms Rachel Still Encountered:
Nights where she would complete a full eight hours yet wake feeling fundamentally unrested, as if sleep had been merely physical without the mental restoration component.

Episodes of waking between 2-4 AM—corresponding with natural cortisol fluctuations—and struggling to return to sleep despite relaxation techniques.

Vivid, stress-themed dreams that reflected her nervous system's continued processing of perceived threats even during rest periods.

Rachel's body had essentially forgotten how to fully surrender to restorative sleep—a pattern that wouldn't spontaneously resolve without specific rehabilitation of normal sleep physiology.

4. Your Relationships Continue to Suffer (Even After You've Changed)

Rachel had made tremendous progress repairing her relationship with Ethan and rebuilding her friendship with Emily, but occasionally still experienced moments of unexpected emotional distance even when genuinely desiring connection.

Why This Happens:
Sustained cortisol exposure increases irritability and reactivity while simultaneously dampening the brain's capacity for empathy and emotional resonance.

Chronic stress significantly reduces activity in brain regions responsible for social connection and emotional attunement to others.

Extended burnout creates habitual emotional withdrawal patterns that persist neurologically even after conscious intentions have changed.

Symptoms Rachel Occasionally Noticed:
Moments of emotional disconnection when she intellectually wanted to be fully present—as if observing interactions from behind an invisible barrier.

Episodes of disproportionate impatience or irritability triggered by minor disruptions, particularly when fatigued.

A subtle but perceptible resistance to deep emotional engagement—a protective detachment that arose without conscious intention.

Rachel was discovering that stress hadn't merely depleted her energy but had fundamentally altered her capacity for connection—requiring deliberate rehabilitation of emotional neural circuits rather than merely improved intentions.

5. Your Aging Accelerates (Your Body Breaks Down Faster Than It Should)

Perhaps most concerning were the physical changes Rachel had begun noticing—subtle shifts in appearance and physical resilience that seemed to have developed rapidly despite her improved lifestyle.

Why This Happens:
Cortisol directly accelerates cellular aging by shortening telomeres—the protective caps on DNA that regulate cell lifespan and function.

Chronic stress systematically degrades collagen production and maintenance, accelerating visible aging, particularly in skin elasticity and appearance.

Prolonged inflammation resulting from stress response creates cumulative cellular damage across multiple body systems, advancing the aging process at the molecular level.

Symptoms Rachel Observed:
Fine lines and skin texture changes that seemed to appear suddenly rather than gradually, particularly during periods of poor sleep.

Slower recovery from minor injuries or illnesses than she had experienced previously.

A general sense of physical fragility or vulnerability that didn't align with her chronological age or overall health status.

These weren't merely aesthetic concerns but visible manifestations of deeper cellular changes resulting from years of hormonal overload—changes that required targeted intervention rather than general wellness practices to address.

How to Start Paying Off Cortisol Debt (Even If You Feel Stuck in Stress Mode)

Confronted with these persistent effects of her years in cortisol debt, Rachel faced a decision point. She could either:

Continue her current approach of stress reduction and hope these lingering symptoms would eventually resolve on their own without specific attention.

Develop a comprehensive rehabilitation plan that directly addresses the collateral damage created by years of hormonal imbalance.

Given the evidence before her—and Dr. Hughes' guidance regarding the persistence of these effects without targeted intervention—she chose deliberate action over passive hope.

What she needed wasn't merely better stress management moving forward but a structured approach to repairing the specific damages her stress addiction had already created.

The Cortisol Debt Payoff Plan — 3 Steps to Escape the Cycle Forever

Rachel had spent years ignoring the accumulating effects of cortisol debt:

She had consistently maxed out her energy credit, pushing beyond sustainable limits through artificial stimulation.

She had borrowed from stress daily, using emergency chemistry to accomplish what should have been managed through sustainable practices.

She had maintained this pattern until her body began implementing forced collection through symptoms she could no longer ignore.

But now, with a clear understanding of both the problem and the solution, she was determined to break the cycle permanently.

No more relying on stress chemistry as functional fuel. No more ignoring the early warning signs of physiological debt. No more paying the compound interest on energy she hadn't actually possessed.

It was time to escape cortisol debt completely—not just temporarily managing symptoms but addressing the root causes that had created her current state.

🔬 Dr. Hughes emphasized that genuine recovery requires more than simply "relaxing more" or adding generic wellness practices to an otherwise unchanged lifestyle.

> "Most recovery attempts fail because people try to add calm without systematically removing stress," he explained during a pivotal session. "They might meditate for ten minutes but spend the rest of the day in fight-or-flight mode. The real solution is three-fold: stop taking on new stress, reset your nervous system fundamentals, and systematically repay what you've borrowed."

The comprehensive three-step process he outlined addressed not just current stress management but the accumulated physiological debt Rachel had developed over years of hormonal overload.

1. Create a "Stress Payoff Budget" (Track & Reduce Cortisol Spikes)

While Rachel had eliminated most major sources of unnecessary stress, she needed a more refined approach to identifying and addressing the subtle cortisol triggers that continued affecting her recovery.

🔬 Dr. Hughes provided a structured formula for this assessment:

Each day, she would document any situation that triggered an identifiable stress response, then evaluate whether that activation represented:

- ☑ **Necessary Challenge (Good for You)** — Situations that create productive engagement without harmful physiological activation, such as meaningful projects, relationship growth opportunities, or beneficial physical exertion.

☒ **Unnecessary Stress (Draining for No Reason)** — Situations creating cortisol elevation without proportional benefit, including manufactured urgency, reflexive people-pleasing, perfectionistic tendencies, or information overload without purpose.

Rachel's systematic tracking revealed an important pattern: While she had successfully eliminated obvious major stressors, subtle but significant triggers remained, particularly around perfectionism in work quality and difficulty declining requests from others, even when clearly unreasonable.

Her goal became complete elimination of these remaining unnecessary stress triggers rather than merely managing their effects.

📝 **Her refined approach included three specific components:**

✅ **Step 1: Identify Hidden Stress Triggers**
Rachel maintained a detailed stress journal for one week, noting every cortisol activation regardless of intensity—including physical sensations, specific triggers, and duration of response.

This meticulous documentation revealed patterns she hadn't previously recognized—including specific people, communication styles, and environments that reliably triggered stress responses.

She identified three particularly significant hidden stressors: perfectionistic revision of already-completed work, difficulty saying no to last-minute requests regardless of their importance, and reflexive checking of work communications during personal time despite no explicit expectation of availability.

✅ **Step 2: Strategic Elimination of Unnecessary Stressors**
Based on this awareness, Rachel implemented specific boundaries around her identified stress triggers:

For perfectionism, she established clear completion criteria before beginning projects and required specific justification for any revisions beyond initial standards.

For boundary issues, she developed templated responses for declining unreasonable requests, removing the need for real-time decision-making when pressure appeared.

For technology management, she created physical separation between work and personal spaces, with work devices remaining in a dedicated location rather than accompanying her throughout her home.

☑ Step 3: Energy Reinvestment

Rather than merely reducing stress, Rachel consciously redirected her reclaimed energy toward recovery activities:

She began treating her energy as finite currency—deliberately allocating it toward priorities rather than allowing it to be claimed by whoever or whatever demanded attention most insistently.

She established "energy profit" targets—specific days when she intentionally ended with more energy than she began, gradually accumulating energy reserves rather than continuing depletion.

By systematically implementing this refined approach, Rachel effectively eliminated virtually all remaining sources of unnecessary cortisol elevation from her daily experience. This comprehensive stress reduction created the essential foundation for addressing the deeper physiological imbalances that persisted from her years of hormonal overload.

2. Reset Your Nervous System (Train Your Body to Exit "Stress Mode")

Despite significant improvements in her conscious stress management, Rachel's nervous system continued occasionally defaulting to emergency response patterns—like a computer continuing to run outdated programming despite software updates.

She needed a complete nervous system recalibration rather than merely improved stress management techniques.

The fundamental misconception most people hold about stress recovery is that it occurs primarily through cognitive change—thinking differently about stressors. While mindset matters, genuine recovery requires direct intervention at the level of the nervous system itself—rewiring physiological responses rather than merely reframing thoughts.

🔬 Dr. Hughes provided Rachel with an advanced three-part protocol specifically designed to reset autonomic nervous system function:

The Expanded Cortisol Flush Protocol

Goal: Reset the nervous system's baseline state from "alert" to "calm" as the default operating condition.

Rachel needed more than occasional stress interruption techniques—she required comprehensive reprogramming of her autonomic nervous system's fundamental settings.

Her enhanced daily protocol included:

- ☑ **Morning nervous system reset:** A structured combination of physiological interventions including brief cold exposure (30-60 second cold shower), specific breathing patterns (extended exhales to trigger parasympathetic activation), and targeted vagus nerve stimulation techniques to signal safety to the nervous system before the day's potential stressors appeared.

- ☑ **Midday pattern interrupt:** Strategically timed breaks specifically calibrated to prevent cortisol accumulation—implemented at 90-minute intervals regardless of work demands to prevent the nervous system from remaining in prolonged activation states.
- ☑ **Evening nervous system downregulation:** A comprehensive approach to signaling safety through environmental cues, including specific light exposure patterns (reducing blue light while increasing amber tones), sound management (white noise or specific frequency sound healing), and temperature regulation (slight cooling to facilitate sleep initiation).

This multifaceted approach effectively forced her nervous system to establish a new operational baseline—one where physiological calm represented the default state rather than requiring special conditions or techniques to achieve.

Through consistent implementation, Rachel's autonomic regulation gradually improved—her nervous system no longer defaulting to emergency mode at the slightest provocation but maintaining relative equilibrium even during legitimate challenges.

The "Pleasure Recalibration" Method

Goal: Retrain the brain's reward circuitry to derive satisfaction from balanced states rather than requiring the intense stimulation of stress chemistry.

Rachel's reward system had been conditioned over years to associate value and satisfaction primarily with high-intensity experiences—the rush of meeting impossible deadlines, the validation of crisis management, the artificial energy of stress-fueled productivity.

To sustain recovery, she needed to recalibrate her pleasure response to recognize and appreciate more balanced physiological states.

Her implementation included:

- ☑ **Daily "flow state" activities** specifically chosen to create focused engagement without stress activation—including painting, creative writing, and musical practice sessions where time disappeared without emergency chemistry.
- ☑ **Strategic dopamine fasting** from artificial sources of stimulation—including scheduled periods completely free from social media, news consumption, and notification-driven technology that had trained her brain to expect constant novel input.
- ☑ **Natural pleasure activation** through evolutionarily aligned experiences—including early morning sunlight exposure, movement in natural settings, and genuine social connection without technological mediation.

This systematic approach effectively retrained her brain's reward circuitry to recognize and value states of balanced engagement rather than requiring the intense but damaging stimulation of stress chemistry for satisfaction.

Rachel gradually began experiencing genuine pleasure in calm, focused activities—breaking her neurological addiction to the intensity of stress-based experiences as the primary source of reward.

The Advanced "Brain Rewire" Protocol

Goal: Permanently alter how the brain processes and responds to potential stressors by creating new neural pathways for stress evaluation.

Even with her significant progress, certain triggers continued activating Rachel's stress response through deeply established neural pathways—automatic reactions that bypassed conscious evaluation.

Lasting change required deliberately creating alternative neural pathways through specific neuroplasticity practices.

Her implementation included:

- ☑ **Deliberate exposure** to mild stressors while maintaining physiological calm—gradually retraining her brain to separate challenge from threat response.
- ☑ **Mental rehearsal** of non-reactive responses to her most common stress triggers—repeatedly visualizing alternative responses until they became more neurologically accessible than her previous stress reactions.
- ☑ **Cognitive reframing** of challenges as growth opportunities rather than threats—a perspective shift reinforced through both intellectual understanding and emotional experience.

This advanced practice utilized neuroplasticity principles to create entirely new neural pathways for processing potentially stressful situations—allowing her brain to evaluate circumstances based on actual threat level rather than conditioned reactivity.

Through consistent implementation of this comprehensive protocol, Rachel's nervous system fundamentally reset—shifting from its previous baseline of hypervigilance and reactivity to a new default state of relative calm punctuated by appropriate, proportional responses to genuine challenges.

3. Add "Recovery Debt Payments" to Your Routine

With unnecessary stressors eliminated and her nervous system returning to healthier function, Rachel faced the final essential component of cortisol debt recovery: deliberately rebuilding her body's depleted energy reserves.

> 🔬 Dr. Hughes emphasized that like financial debt, stress debt requires intentional repayment rather than merely hoping reserves will somehow replenish themselves automatically.

> "Think about it like any significant debt," he explained. "If you've been charging everything to a credit card for years, simply stopping new purchases doesn't eliminate the accumulated balance. You need a deliberate repayment plan with regular contributions toward reducing the principal."

Rachel implemented a structured approach to this energy debt repayment process:

> 📝 **Her daily "recovery debt payments" included three specific components:**
>
> ☑ **Implement Active Recovery (Not Just Passive Rest)**
> Rather than relying on passive downtime like television watching or social media scrolling—activities that often deplete rather than restore energy—Rachel prioritized experiences that actively promote nervous system recovery:
>
> **Nature immersion** became a non-negotiable component of her schedule—including forest bathing practices (mindful time in natural settings) and direct physical contact with natural elements (walking barefoot on earth, swimming in natural bodies of water) that research indicates directly influences nervous system regulation.
>
> **Parasympathetic activation exercises** were implemented throughout her day—including specific breathing patterns, cold exposure, and mechanical vagus nerve stimulation techniques that directly signaled safety to her autonomic nervous system.
>
> **Restorative movement practices** replaced her previous high-intensity exercise patterns—incorporating yoga, tai chi, and gentle swimming that provided physical benefits without triggering stress response.

☑ **Train the Brain to Trust Calmness Again**
Perhaps most challenging was addressing her brain's conditioned distrust of calm states—a common adaptation among high-achievers who have learned to associate stillness with falling behind or missing opportunities.

Rachel systematically retrained this perception:

She practiced periods of "productive stillness"—starting with just five minutes and gradually extending to thirty-minute sessions of simply being present without distraction or activity, directly contradicting her brain's insistence that constant motion was necessary.

Her goal wasn't merely experiencing calm occasionally but making calm feel fundamentally safe—not merely boring, unproductive downtime but a necessary state for optimal function.

She maintained a "calm journal" documenting specific benefits she experienced from these states—creating evidence that directly contradicted her conditioned belief that calm equated to wasted opportunity.

☑ **Rebuild Sleep Architecture with Advanced Recovery Techniques**
Recognizing that sleep quality represented perhaps the most critical factor in true recovery, Rachel implemented a comprehensive protocol for sleep restoration:

Complete digital sunset 2-3 hours before bedtime—eliminating not just blue light but the cognitive and emotional stimulation that accompanies most screen activities.

Bedroom optimization that addressed all sensory aspects of sleep environment—including temperature regulation (maintaining 65-67°F for optimal sleep initiation), complete darkness (blackout curtains, eliminated LED indicators), and sound management (white noise to mask environmental disturbances).

> **Targeted supplementation** to support sleep cycle restoration—including evidence-based compounds like magnesium glycinate for muscle relaxation, L-theanine for mental quieting, and limited CBD use for nervous system regulation when particularly activated.
>
> **Sleep cycle tracking** to ensure she achieved sufficient deep and REM sleep phases—using data to refine her approach rather than merely measuring sleep duration.

Through consistent implementation of these comprehensive recovery practices, Rachel's body gradually rebuilt its depleted energy reserves—transitioning from perpetual deficit to increasing balance and eventually energy surplus.

For the first time in years, she experienced genuine vitality rather than the artificial stimulation of stress hormones or the desperate management of constant fatigue.

Final Takeaway: Pay Off Cortisol Debt Today—Or Your Body Will Force You To

Rachel had experienced firsthand what happens when cortisol debt accumulates without acknowledgment or intervention—the body eventually implements forced collection through increasingly disruptive symptoms that cannot be ignored.

Having developed the tools to address her physiological debt systematically, she had no intention of returning to the patterns that had created her previous condition.

Now equipped with both understanding and practical protocols, she recognized that true freedom from stress involves more than merely managing immediate pressures—it requires fundamental transformation of one's relationship with energy, productivity, and physiological balance.

The same opportunity exists for anyone currently caught in cycles of stress and depletion: The debt can be repaid through deliberate intervention before the body demands payment through illness, breakdown, or collapse.

Once free from cortisol debt, stress no longer controls your biochemistry, energy, or experience—creating genuine autonomy rather than merely better management of chronic depletion.

What Comes Next? Creating a Stress-Free System That Lasts

As Rachel continued implementing her cortisol debt repayment plan, she began experiencing significant improvements in her energy, mental clarity, and overall well-being. The ghost that had haunted her physiology—manifesting through random fatigue crashes, cognitive fog, and unexplained health disruptions—was gradually retreating as she systematically addressed the accumulated effects of years in stress debt.

But as she observed her colleagues at Vertex Media still trapped in cycles of chronic stress and inevitable crashes, a new question emerged:

> Is it enough to just escape burnout personally? Or is there a way to create a life where stress never takes control again?

She was beginning to recognize that true freedom from stress wasn't merely about recovering from past damage but about constructing an entirely different relationship with productivity, achievement, and energy management—creating systems where cortisol debt never accumulates in the first place.

As her body continued healing from years of hormonal overload, her focus expanded toward the next challenge: designing a stress-proof life architecture that would maintain her recovery permanently rather than merely resolving her current symptoms.

And developing that comprehensive stress-prevention system would become her next focus—moving beyond recovery toward genuine transformation of her relationship with stress, achievement, and sustainable performance.

PART III:
THE ESCAPE PLAN

CHAPTER 7: REBUILDING WITHOUT STRESS

Break the Cycle—The Revolutionary Blueprint to Rewire Your Brain and Reclaim Your Life

The Day Success Felt Like Freedom

Rachel stared at her inbox, the blue glow of her monitor casting soft shadows across her face. The numbers displayed in the corner of her screen told a story that would have once triggered an immediate physiological cascade.

23 unread emails. 7 marked "urgent." 3 with red exclamation points.

Six months ago, her response would have been automatic and unquestioned—her heart racing, breathing becoming shallow, shoulders tensing as she prepared to drop everything and address whatever manufactured emergency someone else had deemed critical. She would have canceled lunch plans with Emily, postponed time with Ethan, and surrendered her evening to the insatiable demands of Vertex Media's perpetual urgency.

Today? She simply closed her laptop, the metal surfaces connecting with a soft click that felt like punctuation—the period at the end of a chapter she had finally completed.

The world continued turning on its axis. No clients abandoned ship. No projects imploded. The so-called emergencies resolved themselves or found other paths to completion. The company remained standing despite her choice not to respond with panic.

As she turned away from her desk and walked toward the window, afternoon sunlight warming her face through the glass, a realization crystallized with remarkable clarity—one that would fundamentally reshape her understanding of professional achievement:

> 💬 *What if success was never supposed to hurt? What if everything I've been taught about achievement was a lie? What if the sacrifices I'd made—my energy, my relationships, my health—weren't the price of accomplishment, but simply the cost of doing it wrong?*

The thought expanded through her awareness, rearranging her entire relationship with work and productivity. She had been operating on a fundamental misunderstanding—one that had nearly cost her everything that actually mattered.

💬 *Success without suffering isn't just possible. It's the only kind that lasts.*

Beyond Recovery: When Stress Becomes Irrelevant

Rachel had invested months in transforming her relationship with stress through deliberate, systematic efforts.

She'd methodically broken free from her addiction to urgency, dismantling the neurochemical dependency that had dominated her functioning.

She'd implemented specific protocols to address her accumulated cortisol debt, beginning the process of repaying years of physiological borrowing.

She'd rebuilt her relationship with Ethan through consistent presence and genuine connection, healing what had nearly been lost to her work obsession.

But the state she now found herself in represented something profoundly different from mere improvement or recovery. This wasn't about managing stress better or implementing more effective coping mechanisms. This was about discovering an entirely different mode of human functioning—one where stress wasn't the primary operating system but rather an occasional visitor with diminishing influence.

During her monthly check-in with Dr. Hughes, she attempted to articulate this unfamiliar territory she had entered.

"I can't quite explain it," she said, searching for the right words, "but it's like stress isn't even in the equation anymore. It's not that I'm handling it better—it's that it seems increasingly irrelevant to how I function."

Dr. Hughes nodded with recognition, his expression reflecting both professional satisfaction and genuine pleasure at her progress.

"There's actually a term for what you're experiencing," he explained, leaning forward slightly. "We call it **Stress Immunity**."

"Most people never reach this phase," he continued. "They either remain trapped in cycles of burnout or they develop better stress management without ever transcending it completely. But you've entered the space where stress isn't just controlled—it's becoming progressively irrelevant to your functioning."

Rachel knew exactly what he meant. The transformation wasn't about diminished capabilities or lowered standards. If anything, her capacity had expanded significantly:

Her ability to tackle complex work challenges hadn't decreased with reduced stress—it had sharpened considerably, allowing her to see connections and solutions that had previously been obscured by the fog of constant urgency.

Her problem-solving abilities hadn't suffered from the absence of adrenaline—they had become more sophisticated, nuanced, and effective without the narrowing effect of stress hormones.

Her creative output hadn't declined without the pressure of impossible deadlines—it had flourished in the space created by a calmer nervous system, producing work of greater depth and originality.

But now, these outcomes occurred without the previous costs—no depleted evenings, no weekend recoveries, no relationship sacrifices, no physical symptoms. She was no longer trading pieces of herself for professional accomplishment. The achievement remained while the suffering had been removed from the equation.

Why Most People Struggle to Function Without Stress

🔬 During a particularly insightful session, Dr. Hughes explained that escaping burnout requires more than simply reducing stress—it demands unlearning the deeply ingrained belief that stress is a necessary component of success.

> "For high-achievers especially," he noted, "stress doesn't just feel normal—it feels actively productive. And that association creates perhaps the most challenging aspect of the recovery process."

Rachel nodded, recognizing this pattern in her own experience. For years, she had interpreted the physical and emotional sensations of stress not as warning signs but as indicators she was performing optimally—evidence she was fully engaged and maximally productive.

This represents the fundamental trap that keeps many accomplished professionals locked in stress cycles despite knowing better:

1. The Brain Equates Stress with Motivation

When cortisol and adrenaline levels rise, the brain experiences increased focus and urgency—creating a temporary but powerful enhancement of attention toward whatever has been designated important.

This neurochemical reaction creates a dangerous association between stress activation and productivity—leading people to unconsciously believe they cannot perform effectively without the chemical push that stress hormones provide.

The result becomes a self-reinforcing cycle: people associate their most focused or productive periods with stress activation, creating the impression that stress is a prerequisite for effectiveness rather than a limitation on optimal functioning.

2. Urgency Becomes Addictive

Rachel had grown accustomed to working under conditions of artificial pressure—tight deadlines, crisis management, perpetual motion between urgent tasks. Her nervous system had adapted to this constant stimulation as its baseline operating condition.

Now that her system had reset to calmer functioning, she occasionally experienced an unnerving absence of pressure—moments when the familiar sense of urgency wasn't driving her actions or decisions.

This absence could sometimes create a strange emptiness or restlessness—like a race car driver suddenly finding themselves in a vehicle moving at neighborhood speed limits after years of accelerating around tracks.

The result for many recovering burnout sufferers is unconsciously manufacturing stress where none exists—creating artificial urgency or taking on unnecessary obligations simply to recapture the familiar sensation of pressure that had become comfortable despite its damaging effects.

3. The "Hard Work = Worth" Mindset Runs Deep

Rachel had been raised in a culture that equated effort with value—one that celebrated visible struggle and exhaustion as evidence of character and worth. This conditioning ran deeper than simply professional habits; it formed a core component of her identity and self-concept.

Without the external validation that came from obviously working harder than others, she occasionally questioned her own value and contribution—wondering if her more sustainable approach somehow indicated reduced commitment or dedication.

The result for many high-achievers is sabotaging their own recovery—unconsciously undermining their boundaries or balance because of the uncomfortable feeling that they don't deserve success without visible suffering attached to it.

Through her work with Dr. Hughes, Rachel was learning a profound truth that contradicted everything she had previously believed about performance: The highest level of human functioning doesn't come from pushing harder against limitations—it emerges when the interference of stress chemistry is removed, allowing natural capabilities to express themselves fully without restriction.

Step 1: Rewiring the Brain for Sustainable Success

🔬 During a pivotal session focused on consolidating her progress, Dr. Hughes offered an insight that reframed Rachel's entire approach to improvement.

> "The problem isn't that you need to add more to your system," he explained. "It's that you need to subtract what's getting in the way."

This perspective represented a fundamental shift from how she had previously approached achievement—not as a process of accumulating more techniques, working harder, or pushing beyond limitations, but rather as removing the interference that prevented her natural capabilities from emerging.

To achieve genuinely stress-immune success, Rachel needed to rewire her brain's fundamental understanding of achievement—a process that unfolded through three distinct phases:

Phase 1: Separating Effort from Value
Rachel had unconsciously equated her worth with her level of exhaustion for so long that the connection had become automatic—the more depleted she felt, the more she believed she was contributing meaningfully.

This dangerous association needed to be systematically dismantled through objective evidence rather than theoretical reassurance.

Dr. Hughes provided a simple but powerful daily reflection exercise:

> 1. Document what she actually accomplished each day—specific outcomes and contributions rather than hours worked or effort expended.
> 2. Rate her subjective stress level for the day on a scale of 1-10.
> 3. Analyze the relationship between these variables over time, looking particularly for instances where less stress corresponded with better results.

Within three weeks of consistent documentation, the evidence had become undeniable: her most valuable contributions, most creative solutions, and most effective client interactions consistently occurred on days when her stress levels were lower, not higher.

The data directly contradicted her long-held belief that pressure improved her performance—providing concrete proof that her best work emerged from states of calm focus rather than anxious pushing.

Phase 2: Redefining Productivity
With evidence supporting a new understanding of performance, Rachel completely reimagined what "productivity" actually meant—shifting from quantitative metrics to qualitative ones.

Old definition: Completing numerous tasks quickly regardless of their actual importance or impact; being visibly busy; responding to everything immediately.

New definition: Creating meaningful impact with minimal wasted energy; focusing on high-leverage activities; maintaining clarity amid complexity.

She began measuring her days through entirely different criteria:

Not by hours worked, but by problems elegantly solved with minimal collateral damage.

Not by volume of output, but by clarity of thinking and communication.

Not by exhaustion level at day's end, but by energy remaining for her personal life.

This redefinition fundamentally altered her relationship with productivity—shifting it from a treadmill of constant activity to a thoughtful curation of where her attention and energy would create maximum value.

Phase 3: Experiencing Flow Instead of Force
The culmination of this rewiring process was learning to access flow state consistently—that condition of effortless concentration where time seems to disappear and work feels almost effortless despite high complexity.

Through experimentation, Rachel discovered that flow couldn't be forced through willpower or stress—it emerged reliably only under specific conditions:

Complete focus on a single task without fragmented attention or interruptions.

The absence of stress hormones, which actually prevent the neurological conditions necessary for flow.

Engagement with challenges that matched her skill level—neither too simple (causing boredom) nor too difficult (triggering anxiety).

Clear goals with immediate feedback that allowed continuous adjustment without self-consciousness.

As she systematically created these conditions, Rachel began experiencing extended periods of flow state that previously had been rare occurrences in her work life. The result was counter-intuitive but undeniable—she accomplished more while trying less, experiencing what athletes and artists describe as "the zone" with increasing frequency.

This transformation represented more than better stress management—it was a complete rewiring of how her brain approached work itself, shifting from effortful pushing to aligned engagement that felt simultaneously more effective and less depleting.

Step 2: Rebuilding a Life That Felt Alive

Rachel had spent years in survival mode—moving from one deadline to the next, one crisis to another, maintaining professional function at the cost of genuine living. She had become so accustomed to mere existence that the possibility of actual thriving seemed almost foreign.

Now, she wanted to start living, not just surviving—but where do you begin when you've ignored joy for so long?

> During a session focused on this next phase of development, Dr. Hughes introduced a concept that expanded her thinking beyond stress management to genuine vitality.

"Think of your life as an energy ecosystem," he suggested, sketching a simple diagram on his notepad. "Some activities inevitably drain you—that's unavoidable. Others merely sustain you—keeping you functioning without depletion. But a select few actually generate new energy—creating more vitality than they consume."

He looked up, meeting her eyes directly. "Stress immunity requires more than just avoiding burnout—it demands the regular inclusion of activities that actively generate energy rather than merely conserve it."

This framework provided Rachel with a clear structure for rebuilding a life characterized by vitality rather than mere absence of exhaustion:

1. **Identify Energy Generators**

Rachel methodically catalogued activities that consistently left her with more energy than when she started—experiences that created genuine vitality rather than consuming it:

Early morning walks in nature, particularly as sunrise transformed the city park near her apartment.

Creative writing without deadlines or expectations—simply following her thoughts wherever they led.

Deep, unhurried conversations with Ethan, where she discovered who he was becoming rather than merely managing logistics.

Playing piano—an activity she had abandoned years earlier when "productivity" became her sole focus.

She committed to incorporating at least one energy-generating activity daily without exception—treating these not as optional luxuries but as essential investments in her core vitality.

2. **Minimize Energy Drains**

Next, she ruthlessly evaluated what consistently depleted her energy without providing proportional value—the activities that created net energy deficits without sufficient return:

Meetings that could have been handled through brief written communication.

People-pleasing responses that committed her to activities misaligned with her priorities.

Perfectionism applied to low-impact areas where "good enough" would suffice.

Mindless consumption of news and social media left her depleted rather than informed or connected.

She systematically eliminated or contained these activities, implementing specific boundaries around unavoidable energy drains while completely removing optional ones.

3. Design Energy Net Positive Days

With a clear understanding of what generated versus depleted her energy, Rachel restructured her daily patterns to ensure she consistently ended days with more vitality than she began them:

Energy-generating activities were positioned early in her day, creating immediate vitality deposits before withdrawals began.

Her most demanding work was scheduled during her natural energy peaks rather than pushed into periods of typical depletion.

Energy-neutral activities (those neither notably depleting nor energizing) were clustered during predictable low points in her natural energy rhythm.

She limited herself to a maximum of two significant energy-draining activities per day, regardless of external pressure.

The result of this systematic approach was transformative. For the first time in her adult life,

Rachel consistently finished days feeling energized rather than depleted—experiencing a cumulative increase in vitality rather than the progressive exhaustion that had previously characterized her existence.

She wasn't merely avoiding burnout anymore—she was actively generating vitality through deliberate energy management.

Step 3: Making Sure This Lasts Forever

Through her recovery journey, Rachel had learned a crucial principle: balance isn't a static achievement but a dynamic process requiring continuous attention and adjustment. Without vigilance, old patterns could gradually reassert themselves, eroding progress before she fully recognized their return.

To prevent this regression, she needed more than good intentions—she required a systematic approach to maintaining her transformed relationship with stress, productivity, and energy.

She created a comprehensive system to protect her new approach—establishing non-negotiable protocols that would prevent stress from regaining control of her life.

Rachel's Stress Immunity Protocol:

1. **The Energy ROI Rule**
Rachel developed a consistent filter through which every potential commitment had to pass—a deliberate evaluation of its energy return on investment:

Will this activity or commitment ultimately generate more energy than it requires?

If not, is it genuinely necessary rather than merely expected or habitual?

If both necessary and potentially depleting, how can its impact be contained to prevent broader energy drain?

This single decision-making framework eliminated approximately 80% of potential stress triggers before they could enter her life—creating a protective boundary that filtered commitments based on their actual impact rather than superficial urgency.

2. **The Recovery-First Calendar**
Rather than following the conventional approach of scheduling work commitments and attempting to fit recovery around them, Rachel deliberately inverted this process:

Essential recovery periods were blocked in her calendar first—non-negotiable appointments with activities that generated rather than depleted energy.

Work commitments were then arranged around these protected blocks rather than automatically taking precedence over them.

Perhaps most importantly, these recovery periods were treated as immovable—not subject to sacrifice for "emergencies" regardless of how urgent they might appear.

This calendar approach ensured that recovery wasn't merely theoretical but actually integrated into her daily reality—protected space for energy renewal rather than an aspiration consistently sacrificed to immediate demands.

3. The Quarterly Life Audit

Recognizing that systems tend to drift without regular recalibration, Rachel established a formal review process every three months—a comprehensive evaluation of her entire stress immunity system:

Was stress beginning to reappear in subtle ways? Where specifically, and through what mechanisms?

Had new energy drains developed that weren't being adequately addressed?

Had her definition of success subtly shifted back toward struggle rather than sustainable achievement?

She approached these reviews with the same seriousness she had previously applied to professional evaluations—treating them as essential maintenance rather than optional reflection.

The combined effect of these systematic safeguards was a self-reinforcing cycle of sustainable performance—one that actively prevented regression while continuously refining her approach to success without stress.

She wasn't merely experiencing temporary relief from burnout—she had designed a life where the patterns leading to burnout had become structurally impossible rather than simply avoided.

The Freedom Beyond Recovery

One evening as twilight settled over the city, Rachel sat on her apartment balcony with a glass of wine, listening to a piece of music she'd never had time to truly hear before. The complex interplay of instruments washed over her as the last light faded from the sky and city lights began emerging like earthbound stars.

There were no looming deadlines demanding her attention. Her thoughts moved at their natural pace rather than racing ahead to the next obligation. The perpetual pull of stress that had once fragmented her attention into a thousand pieces had quieted, allowing her to be fully present in this single, ordinary moment.

Her phone vibrated against the small table beside her. In the past, that sound would have triggered an immediate response—an almost Pavlovian reach for the device, regardless of what it might be interrupting.

Tonight, she glanced at it with mild curiosity rather than compulsive urgency.

Emily: *"What's the plan for tomorrow?"*

Rachel considered the question, realizing it no longer created the familiar tension of needing to optimize every moment, to have everything structured and controlled.

Rachel: *"No plan. Just living."*

Those four simple words represented the culmination of her transformation—not merely a temporary absence of obligations but a fundamental shift in how she engaged with life itself.

She had built an existence where stress wasn't just managed better or temporarily held at bay—it had become largely irrelevant to her daily experience, an occasional visitor rather than the dominating force it had once been.

And in that space beyond stress addiction, beyond cortisol debt, beyond the perpetual push for more, she had discovered something unexpected—not emptiness or reduced achievement, but genuine freedom.

Redefining What "Hard Work" Actually Means

Throughout her career, Rachel had operated under a set of unexamined assumptions about the relationship between effort and success:

More hours automatically translate to greater productivity and value. More stress indicates deeper dedication and commitment. More exhaustion at the end of the day represents greater contribution.

But she had discovered through direct experience that these equations were fundamentally flawed.

Dr. Hughes helped her understand that genuine high performance isn't about quantity of effort but quality of engagement—not how much you work but how effectively you direct your energy.

> "The most accomplished people in any field aren't distinguished by their capacity for suffering," he explained during a session focused on sustainable achievement. "They're distinguished by their ability to eliminate everything that interferes with their natural capabilities—including the stress that most people mistake for productivity."

This insight led Rachel to develop a new framework for understanding genuine productivity:

1. Time Spent ≠ Productivity

> *Success isn't measured by hours invested but by value created—what you accomplish during those hours, rather than simply accumulating them.*

This principle was demonstrated whenever Rachel completed in two focused hours what previously might have taken an entire distracted, stress-filled day—evidence that duration of effort correlates poorly with actual output.

2. Urgency ≠ Importance

> 💡 *The perceived pressure associated with a task rarely correlates with its actual significance—many genuinely important responsibilities generate no urgency signals at all.*

Rachel observed this reality whenever she compared what felt pressing in the moment with what actually created lasting impact—recognizing that the tasks screaming loudest for attention were rarely those that mattered most.

3. Exhaustion ≠ Worth

> 💡 *Value isn't measured by depletion but by contribution—your significance doesn't depend on how drained you feel at day's end.*

This truth became evident as Rachel's most meaningful professional contributions increasingly came on days when she maintained energy throughout rather than depleting herself completely.

Through these realigned principles, Rachel developed a fundamentally different relationship with productivity—one based on effectiveness rather than suffering, on meaningful impact rather than visible struggle.

She was learning that genuine success didn't require breaking herself in the process—it actually emerged most consistently when she maintained her wholeness and vitality rather than sacrificing them on the altar of achievement.

Converting Chaos into Calm: The Alchemist's Approach

As Rachel's transformation deepened, she discovered something extraordinary about her relationship with challenge and difficulty. While those around her continued responding to unexpected problems with stress and urgency, she had developed the capacity to approach the same situations with a fundamentally different mindset.

During one of their sessions, Dr. Hughes articulated what he was observing in her evolution:

"Most people see chaos as something to be endured—a storm to weather until calm returns. But you're developing something far more valuable—the ability to transmute chaos itself, to find opportunity in the very situations others experience as threatening."

This capacity was tested dramatically during a presentation to Vertex's most significant client—a meeting where Rachel was scheduled to present critical strategic recommendations to their executive team.

Ten minutes before her presentation began, the projector failed completely. The backup system was quickly deployed but exhibited the same malfunction. Her colleagues immediately entered crisis mode—frantic calls to technical support, desperate attempts to transfer files to alternative devices, voices rising with tension as the client team waited in the conference room.

The Rachel of six months earlier would have joined this collective panic, absorbing and amplifying the stress of the situation. Her nervous system would have interpreted the technical failure as a personal emergency requiring fight-or-flight activation.

The Rachel who stood calmly observing the situation now did something entirely different.

She sat down quietly at the conference table, momentarily separating herself from the frantic activity around her. She observed the chaos without absorbing its energy, maintaining her own physiological equilibrium despite the external disorder.

Rather than responding reactively from a place of stress, she thought strategically from a position of calm clarity—considering what the situation offered rather than focusing solely on what had been lost.

After a moment of reflection, she stood up with quiet authority.

"We don't need slides," she announced, her voice composed enough to cut through the anxious chatter. "Let's rearrange into a circle and have a conversation instead. I'd rather hear your questions and concerns directly than present to you anyway."

The energy in the room shifted palpably as chairs were rearranged from the traditional presentation format into a more intimate circular configuration. What had moments before been experienced as a technical disaster transformed into something unexpected—one of the most engaging and productive client interactions they had conducted all year.

The absence of slides eliminated the barrier of formality, allowing genuine dialogue about the client's underlying concerns rather than merely addressing what had been prepared in advance. The conversation revealed priorities and perspectives that might never have emerged in a standard presentation format.

When the meeting concluded successfully, her director approached her with undisguised amazement.

"How did you stay so calm when everything went wrong?" he asked, clearly trying to understand what he had witnessed.

Rachel smiled, recognizing how foreign her response must appear to someone still operating from the stress-based paradigm she had left behind.

"I realized a while ago that most disasters aren't actually disasters," she explained. "They're invitations to innovation that we miss when we're too busy panicking to see the opportunity they present."

In that moment, she recognized she had mastered something few professionals ever develop: the ability to see chaos not as a threat requiring emergency response but as raw material waiting to be transformed through calm presence and creative engagement.

The Turning Point: Success Without Struggle

On a crisp autumn afternoon, Rachel met with Emily at their usual café—the familiar environment highlighting how significantly her internal landscape had changed since they had begun meeting there during her early recovery.

Emily studied her friend with the unique perspective of someone who had witnessed her entire journey—from stress addiction through burnout to her current state of unusual equilibrium.

"I can't quite put my finger on it," Emily observed, stirring her latte thoughtfully, "but you're... operating on a different level now. It's like watching someone who's found a shortcut the rest of us don't know exists."

Rachel considered this assessment as she sipped her tea, recognizing its accuracy. "I'm just not fighting myself anymore," she replied, realizing how fundamental this shift had been.

The transformation wasn't merely about better stress management techniques or improved boundaries. It represented a complete recalibration of her relationship with achievement itself:

She no longer experienced the perpetual sense of being overwhelmed that had once seemed an inevitable companion to accomplishment.

The constant state of energy depletion that she had mistaken for dedication had been replaced by sustainable vitality.

Perhaps most significantly, she had stopped measuring her professional worth by how exhausted she felt—recognizing this as a fundamentally flawed metric of contribution.

For the first time in her professional life, she was working with her natural energy patterns rather than constantly forcing herself to override them—discovering that alignment produced better results with substantially less effort than perpetual pushing had ever achieved.

Can You Handle Pressure Without Burning Out?

The ultimate test of Rachel's transformation wasn't how she functioned during periods of relative calm but how she responded when genuine pressure appeared—whether she could maintain her new operating system when circumstances might easily trigger reversion to familiar stress patterns.

Rachel had fundamentally changed her relationship with work and achievement:

She no longer depended on stress chemistry as motivational fuel for productivity.

She had learned to work effectively without the artificial urgency that once drove her actions. She had established and maintained genuine boundaries that protected her wellbeing.

But these changes would face inevitable challenges, because regardless of her personal transformation, certain realities remained unchanged:

Deadlines still existed and sometimes clustered together unavoidably. Difficult personalities and challenging interactions remained part of professional life. Unexpected complexities and genuine crises occasionally emerged, requiring immediate attention.

The question wasn't whether she could escape stress entirely—an unrealistic aspiration in a complex world—but whether she could engage with legitimate pressure without reverting to the burnout patterns that had previously dominated her life.

Rachel had mastered escaping unnecessary stress. Now she needed to develop the capacity to handle necessary pressure without allowing it to trigger the dysfunctional responses she had worked so diligently to transform.

Step 1: Changing the Default Stress Response

Rachel discovered that true transformation wasn't about managing stress better—it was about rewiring her automatic responses completely.

During their work together, Dr. Hughes introduced her to the concept of "response pathways"—the neural circuits that form through repeated patterns of reaction, eventually becoming automatic rather than conscious choices.

"Your brain has developed a well-worn path from trigger to stress reaction," he explained, sketching a simple diagram showing how neural connections strengthen through repetition. "Each time you respond to pressure with your stress addiction behaviors, you reinforce that pathway. Our job is to create and strengthen an entirely new response sequence."

The opportunity to test this new pathway arrived unexpectedly during a high-stakes client presentation. Rachel had prepared extensively for the meeting, but shortly after she began, the client's CEO interrupted with a series of aggressive questions that directly challenged core elements of her strategy.

The room grew uncomfortably silent as everyone turned to observe her response. Colleagues who had witnessed similar situations before expected her to either become defensively rigid or accommodatingly flustered—the typical polarized reactions to public challenge.

Her body's initial response followed familiar patterns—a tightening sensation in her chest, increased heart rate, a surge of defensive energy preparing her nervous system for confrontation.

But instead of being hijacked by these sensations, Rachel observed them with curious awareness—noting their presence without allowing them to determine her response.

> 💬 *Interesting. My body's preparing for threat. But this isn't actually threatening—it's an opportunity for greater clarity.*

She took a deliberate breath, slightly lengthening her exhale, and smiled genuinely rather than defensively.

"Those are excellent questions," she acknowledged, her voice steady and engaged rather than stressed or apologetic. "They highlight precisely where we need more precision in our approach. Let's explore each concern in detail."

For the next twenty minutes, she led the room through a methodical examination of the questions raised, transforming what could have been confrontational into collaborative problem-solving that ultimately strengthened rather than undermined the proposed strategy.

When the meeting concluded successfully, a colleague approached her with barely concealed amazement. "How did you stay so composed? I would have completely panicked facing that level of challenge."

Rachel realized something profound had changed in her operating system. The previously automatic pathway from trigger to stress response had been replaced with an entirely new sequence:

Trigger → Awareness → Choice → Strategic Response

This wasn't merely better stress management through willpower. It represented fundamental rewiring of her default reactions—creating new neural pathways that would eventually become as automatic as her previous stress responses had been.

Her default setting was no longer panic but presence—not through constant effort but through reconditioning her most basic responses to pressure.

Step 2: Learning to Work Under Pressure—Without Overworking

Throughout her career, Rachel had unconsciously equated stress with increased output—believing that pressure demanded overperformance as its natural and necessary response.

Deadlines had automatically triggered longer hours, skipped meals, and sleep sacrifice. Challenging projects had justified boundary violations and relationship neglect. High-stakes situations demanded entry into crisis mode regardless of whether emergency functioning improved outcomes.

But stress was never actually the source of her effectiveness—it was merely the fuel she had habitually employed, often at tremendous cost to her well-being and relationships.

Now she needed to develop a better fuel source—a way to perform effectively under genuine pressure without triggering the dysfunctional patterns that had previously characterized her response to challenge.

The "Slow Down to Speed Up" Strategy

🔬 Drawing from research in performance psychology, Dr. Hughes introduced Rachel to a counter-intuitive principle: high performers actually work more effectively when they deliberately slow down under pressure rather than accelerating.

> "This seems paradoxical until you understand the neurophysiology," he explained. "When the brain perceives urgency, it activates survival-based functioning—which is extraordinarily effective for escaping predators but remarkably poor for complex cognitive tasks."

The science revealed several important mechanisms:

> When experiencing pressure, the brain naturally activates survival circuitry that prioritizes speed over accuracy, immediate response over strategic consideration, and familiar patterns over creative solutions.
>
> This activation creates the illusion of productivity through increased activity levels, but typically results in more errors, poorer decisions, and ultimately greater time investment to correct problems created through hasty responses.
>
> Deliberately slowing down during pressure situations allows maintained access to higher brain functions—particularly the prefrontal cortex responsible for executive function, strategic thinking, and creative problem-solving.

Understanding these principles, Rachel developed a deliberate practice of doing exactly the opposite of what pressure seemed to demand:

When deadlines loomed, she intentionally slowed her pace and created more space for reflective thinking rather than accelerating into frantic activity.

When complex problems arose, she deliberately paused to consider multiple approaches rather than immediately implementing the first solution that appeared.

When situations felt urgent, she reminded herself of the fundamental principle: "Pressure doesn't mean panic—it means presence is even more important."

The results of this counter-intuitive approach consistently surprised her. By consciously slowing down rather than speeding up under pressure, she completed projects with fewer errors requiring correction, made better strategic decisions, and ultimately accomplished more meaningful work in less time than her previous stress-based approach had ever achieved.

She was effectively handling the same workload and meeting the same deadlines—but with half the stress and significantly better outcomes. This represented a fundamental revision of her relationship with pressure—transforming it from a trigger for dysfunction into a signal for heightened presence and deliberate engagement.

This was how sustainable success became possible—not through avoiding all pressure, but through responding to it in ways that enhanced rather than compromised effectiveness.

How to Use Stress Without Letting It Use You

For years, Rachel had conceptualized stress exclusively as her enemy—something to be avoided, overcome, or escaped at all costs. She had fought against it, attempted to eliminate it completely, and viewed it as the primary destructive force that had nearly demolished her health, relationships, and well-being.

But as her recovery deepened, a more nuanced understanding began emerging—one that recognized stress wasn't inherently destructive in all forms and contexts. The problem had never been stress itself but rather how she had engaged with it: its chronic nature, her lack of recovery periods, and her inability to maintain perspective during pressure situations.

This evolving perspective shifted her fundamental question from:
💬 *"How do I completely eliminate stress from my life?"*

To the more sophisticated inquiry:
💬 *"How do I use certain aspects of stress response constructively without allowing them to control me?"*

This represented a significant evolution in her relationship with pressure—moving from avoidance to mastery, from victim to director of her own physiological responses.

The Science of "Good" Stress vs. "Toxic" Stress

🔬 In exploring this more nuanced approach, Dr. Hughes helped Rachel understand the crucial scientific distinction between different types of stress response and their dramatically different impacts on human functioning.

> "Stress itself isn't inherently harmful," he explained during a session focused on this advanced perspective. "In fact, certain forms of stress are necessary for growth, development, and optimal performance. The problem isn't stress per se—it's chronic stress without adequate recovery."

The research revealed important distinctions:

- ☑ **Good Stress (Eustress):** Brief, contained periods of stress that create positive adaptation when followed by sufficient recovery—similar to how appropriate exercise stresses muscles to stimulate growth provided adequate rest follows.
- ☑ **Toxic Stress (Chronic Stress):** Extended periods of stress without adequate recovery that create progressive damage to physical systems, cognitive function, and emotional well-being.

Rachel had spent the majority of her professional life immersed in toxic stress patterns—maintaining chronic activation without recovery periods, essentially treating a sprint as if it were a sustainable pace for a marathon.

Now she was developing the capacity to engage with good stress in appropriate contexts and durations—utilizing the focused attention and heightened engagement that short-term stress can facilitate without allowing it to become a chronic condition.

Step 3: Setting a "Stress Threshold"

Rachel recognized that while she had transformed her relationship with stress, she needed clear parameters to maintain this change—specific boundaries beyond which she would not allow pressure to push her regardless of circumstances.

She established a stress threshold—a personal limit that would serve as an early warning system long before burnout could begin developing again.

Rachel's New Stress Limits:

1. If she felt stress rising, she had to stop and ask: "Is this actually my problem?"

> 💡 *No more automatically absorbing responsibility for issues that properly belonged to others—a pattern that had previously expanded her stress load exponentially.*

2. If her sleep or energy started declining, she had to adjust immediately.

> 💡 *No more ignoring physiological warning signs until they escalate into full burnout symptoms.*

3. If she felt overwhelmed, she had to drop the least important task first.

> 💡 Not everything requires immediate completion, regardless of how urgent it might appear.

These thresholds created automatic protective responses that activated long before stress could accumulate to harmful levels.

How to Make Sure Stress Never Takes Over Again

Rachel had established a life where unnecessary stress had been systematically eliminated. Now she needed to ensure these changes endured permanently rather than eventually eroding under future pressures.

Step 1: The "Never Again" List

Rachel created a formal documentation of lines she would not cross under any circumstances:

- ☑ I will never let stress determine my worth.
- ☑ I will never take on responsibilities that aren't mine.
- ☑ I will never sacrifice sleep for work.
- ☑ I will never say yes to things that drain me without proportional value.
- ☑ I will never ignore my body's warning signs again.

This wasn't merely a temporary motivation tool but a contract with herself—explicit parameters that would remain in force regardless of how circumstances evolved.

Step 2: The "Quarterly Burnout Check-In"

To ensure consistent maintenance rather than gradual erosion, Rachel established a formal quarterly review process:

Every 90 days, she systematically assessed:

1. Am I feeling drained or energized by my work?
2. Am I still protecting my personal time, or am I letting work creep in?

3. Am I making decisions based on alignment, or out of obligation?
4. Am I still saying no to things that don't serve me?
5. Is my success still sustainable—or am I slipping into old patterns?

If these assessments revealed concerning patterns, she committed to immediate correction rather than postponing adjustment.

Step 3: Having a Burnout Exit Plan—Before It's Needed

Despite her comprehensive prevention systems, Rachel created specific response protocols before they might be needed:

Rachel's Burnout Exit Plan:

1. **If I feel burnout symptoms, I will take action within 24 hours.**
   💡 *No waiting for "better timing" or hoping problems will resolve spontaneously.*

2. **If my work-life balance starts slipping, I will reassess all commitments.**
   💡 *Examining the full landscape of obligations rather than focusing exclusively on obvious pressure points.*

3. **If stress becomes overwhelming, I will step back before it escalates.**
   💡 *Creating space for assessment and recalibration rather than continuing engagement under suboptimal conditions.*

The Quiet Permanence of Peace

One evening as twilight settled over the city, Rachel sat on her balcony, watching the sunset paint the sky in deepening hues. No urgent work demands competed for her attention. No digital notifications interrupted her awareness. No subtle guilt about "wasting time" contaminated her enjoyment.

Her phone vibrated. She glanced at the screen without urgency.

 Emily: *"Do you ever miss the old version of yourself?"*

After a moment of genuine reflection, she typed her response:

Rachel: *"Not even a little."*

She had constructed a life where stress no longer determined her worth, dictated her choices, or dominated her experience. She had transformed her fundamental relationship with achievement, pressure, and her own value.

And this time, it was forever.

What Comes Next? Deepening the Practice When Challenges Strike

Rachel had created systems to protect her energy, reconfigured her work approach, and redefined success on her own terms. But as she looked around at her colleagues still trapped in burnout culture, she wondered:

💬 *Is my transformation strong enough to withstand a real crisis?*

True freedom wasn't just about changing daily habits—it was about developing practices that could withstand life's inevitable storms. What would happen when a genuine emergency demanded her attention? When life threw her a challenge that couldn't be delegated or postponed?

She needed a methodology for maintaining her cortisol balance even in the face of genuine pressure.

And learning to master cortisol fasting would be her next challenge.

CHAPTER 8: CORTISOL FASTING

Fasting from Stress—How I Survived Collapse and Turned My Nervous System Into an Ally

The Day Rachel's World Caught Fire

Rachel had spent months learning how to live without stress. She had mastered staying calm under pressure.

She had built systems to maintain her energy balance.

She had finally escaped burnout's relentless grip, transforming her work and life. She thought she was untouchable.

But then, the letter arrived.

A single sheet of paper—stamped, official, cold—that threatened to undo everything she had built.

Legal Notice: Petition for Full Custody

Her heart stopped as the words registered. Michael, her ex-husband, was trying to take Ethan away.

Rachel stared at the document, feeling the familiar tightness beginning in her chest. After everything she'd learned, after all the work she'd done to transform herself, her past was coming back to haunt her in the most devastating way possible.

This wasn't just any challenge. This was Ethan—the relationship that mattered most. And for the first time since her recovery, she faced a threat that could genuinely push her back into the stress spiral she had fought so hard to escape.

Why Now? Why Him? Why This?

Michael had always been in the background of her life. Their divorce three years earlier had been relatively civil despite the tensions. He had received primary custody given Rachel's demanding work schedule at the time, but she had maintained meaningful involvement in Ethan's life, especially as she rebuilt herself in recent months.

Their arrangement wasn't perfect, but it had been working. Until now.

One paragraph in the document stood out with painful clarity:

"The petitioner submits that respondent Rachel Summers has demonstrated consistent patterns of instability, chronic stress, and emotional unavailability that make her unfit for continued shared custody. Respondent has historically prioritized professional obligations above parental responsibilities, resulting in a pattern of neglect that has negatively impacted the minor child's emotional development."

But it was the final sentence that turned her blood cold:

"Petitioner has documented evidence supporting these claims."

The cruel irony wasn't lost on her. Michael wasn't making empty accusations. He was using her past—the burned-out, stress-addicted, emotionally absent mother she had been—as a weapon against the person she had fought to become.

Every missed school event, every canceled weekend, every distracted conversation with Ethan while she checked emails—Michael had been keeping track. And now, just when she had finally transformed herself, he was using who she used to be to take away what mattered most.

The Weaponized Past

Rachel spread the documents across her kitchen counter. Beyond the initial petition was a detailed catalog of her shortcomings as a mother—each incident meticulously dated and described.

June 15, 2022: Missed Ethan's end-of-year school play despite six weeks' advance notice. Text message from respondent at 5:17 PM stating "emergency client situation" prevented attendance.

October 28, 2022: Scheduled weekend with minor child canceled with less than 24 hours' notice due to "work deadline." Third such cancellation within a two-month period.

March 4, 2023: Observed checking emails repeatedly during parent-teacher conference, asking the teacher to repeat information multiple times due to inattention. Teacher noted child's visible disappointment.

Page after page, she documented moments when she had failed Ethan—when work had taken precedence, when burnout had stolen her presence, and when stress had made her a shadow in her son's life rather than a supportive presence.

The most painful part wasn't the accusations themselves—it was their fundamental truth. She couldn't deny a single incident. Each one had happened exactly as described, a perfect record of the mother she had been during her worst burnout periods.

For years, she had been exactly the mother Michael claimed she was: distracted, overwhelmed, and physically present but mentally elsewhere.

The legal document might as well have been written in her own blood—Michael was using her authentic failings, her genuine mistakes, to portray her as someone she no longer was. The evidence wasn't fabricated; it was simply outdated. Yet in a legal proceeding, would that distinction matter?

The Return of Cortisol: How Stress Tries to Take Control

Dr. Hughes had warned her that this would happen.

"Recovery isn't linear," he had explained during one of their sessions months earlier. "You'll experience moments where significant stressors threaten to pull you back into old patterns. That's not failure—it's the inevitable testing of new neural pathways."

But theoretical understanding offered little comfort as Rachel felt her body's visceral response—the cascade of stress hormones flooding her system despite her conscious desire to remain calm.

Within moments of reading the custody petition, her carefully reconstructed equilibrium began to unravel. Her heart hammered against her ribs with a force that seemed to shake her entire body. Her breathing shortened to rapid, shallow gasps that left her light-headed. Her vision narrowed as her brain directed all resources to the perceived threat, the edges of her kitchen blurring as she focused only on the papers before her.

The physical sensations were distressingly familiar—the same biochemical cascade that had characterized her years at Vertex Media, the same fight-or-flight activation that had eventually led to her breakdown. But now, the stakes felt immeasurably higher. This wasn't about a client deadline or a marketing emergency.

This was about her son.

Her mind raced with fragmented thoughts:
💬 *I need to call a lawyer immediately.*
💬 *I should confront Michael directly.*
💬 *What if I lose Ethan completely?*
💬 *How could he do this now, just when I've finally changed?*

Each thought triggered fresh panic, each wave of fear generating more fragmented thinking. The recursive loop threatened to pull her into exactly the stress-driven reactivity that had characterized her previous life—the very patterns she had spent months dismantling.

The realization hit her with surprising clarity even through the biochemical storm: This was the moment that would determine whether her transformation was merely situational or genuinely fundamental. The true test wasn't whether she could avoid stress triggers—it was whether she could maintain her new operating system when those triggers inevitably appeared.

As the cortisol surged through her body, Rachel faced a critical choice:

Would she surrender to the neurochemical cascade, allowing stress to reclaim control?

Or would she implement the systems she had built, proving that her transformation went beyond theory into genuine resilience?

She chose the second option.

Step 1: The Emergency Cortisol Fast

Rachel knew she had two options.

She could spiral into stress, make rash decisions, and lose control—exactly what Michael's petition was designed to provoke.

Or she could use the system she had spent months building—to shut the stress down before it destroyed her clarity.

🔬 The Emergency Cortisol Fast wasn't just about calming down—it was about actively resetting her nervous system at the neurochemical level. Dr. Hughes had designed this protocol specifically for moments when typical stress management wouldn't be enough.

> ☑ She deliberately turned off her phone, silencing the temptation to make reactive calls or send emotional messages. The custody petition remained on the counter while she stepped.
>
> First, she needed to stop feeding the stress response.
>
> away from it—physically creating distance from the trigger. She closed her laptop, eliminating the possibility of sending a hasty email she might regret.
>
> "No immediate responses," she murmured to herself, recalling Dr. Hughes' guidance. "Not while the chemistry is controlling my thinking."
>
> The next step required something more dramatic.
>
> ☑ Walking to her bathroom, Rachel turned the shower to its coldest setting. Without giving herself time to reconsider, she stepped under the icy stream, gasping as the shock of cold water hit her skin.

The effect was immediate and profound—her body couldn't maintain its stress response while simultaneously adapting to the temperature change.

> The cold exposure forced an automatic physiological shift, activating the parasympathetic nervous system that counterbalanced the fight-or-flight response that had been dominating her system. The scientific term was "mammalian dive reflex"—an evolutionary mechanism that overrides stress activation when the body encounters cold water.

After ninety seconds, Rachel stepped out of the shower, her skin tingling and her breathing significantly deeper. The panic hadn't disappeared completely, but its grip had loosened enough to allow clearer thinking.

Still dripping, she wrapped herself in a towel and reached for the notebook she kept beside her bed. Opening to a blank page, she wrote a single question:

💬 *What is the next logical step? Not emotional—logical?*

> ☑ The act of writing engaged her prefrontal cortex—the brain region responsible for rational thought and executive function, the very region that stress chemistry tends to bypass in favor of more reactive systems.
>
> By deliberately activating this area through writing, she was creating a pathway back to strategic thinking rather than emotional reactivity.

The cortisol was still present in her system, but it no longer controlled her response. She had created enough space between stimulus and reaction to choose her path forward deliberately.

This wasn't just stress management. This was stress mastery—the ability to experience the physiological response without surrendering to its control.

The First Move in the Battle

Rachel sat at her kitchen table with the custody petition arranged neatly before her. The emergency reset protocol had done its job—her hands no longer trembled, her breathing had returned to normal depths, and most importantly, her thinking had shifted from chaotic panic to focused problem-solving.

☑ She reached for her phone and typed a message to Emily:

Rachel to Emily: *"I need a lawyer. Now."*

The simplicity of the text belied the complexity of thought behind it. She wasn't asking for emotional support or venting her panic—she was taking concrete, strategic action to address the threat facing her. This wasn't the stress-addicted Rachel reacting to crisis; this was the transformed Rachel responding with clarity.

Emily's reply came almost immediately:

Emily: *"On it."*

While waiting for Emily's next message, Rachel began methodically reviewing the custody petition, notebook beside her to document key points requiring response. Each accusation that once might have triggered defensive emotion was now categorized, analyzed, and evaluated for strategy rather than reaction.

> *Michael isn't just challenging my legal rights*, but she realized that patterns emerged from the document. *He's challenging my entire transformation—using who I was to erase who I've become.*

This wasn't merely a legal proceeding. This was a referendum on whether people could truly change—whether past mistakes could be overcome through genuine transformation, or whether they remained permanent definitions of character regardless of growth.

Her phone vibrated with Emily's follow-up:

Emily: *"Catherine Reyes. Best family law attorney in the city. She can see you tomorrow at 9 AM. I'll text you her office address."*

Rachel exhaled slowly, feeling the steadying effect of concrete action replacing helpless anxiety. She had a direction now, a first step in what would undoubtedly be a challenging process.

📩 **Rachel to Emily:** *"Thank you. I owe you."*

📩 **Emily:** *"You owe me nothing. Just keep breathing."*

Those three words—*just keep breathing*—struck Rachel with unexpected force. They weren't mere comfort but recognition of how fundamentally her approach to crisis had changed. Six months ago, breathing would have been the last thing on her mind during an emergency. Now it was the first.

She closed her eyes briefly, feeling the gentle rise and fall of her chest, the steady rhythm that anchored her to the present moment rather than catastrophic future scenarios. Each breath represented a choice—to remain in this moment rather than being hijacked by panic about what might happen.

Tomorrow would bring legal consultation and strategy. Tonight required continued stability—maintaining the physiological equilibrium she had fought so hard to establish.

Why Cortisol Fasting Is the Key to Winning High-Stakes Battles

"So Michael has essentially been building a case against me for years," Rachel explained to Dr. Hughes during their scheduled session. "Using my past behavior to argue that I'm fundamentally unfit as a mother."

"And how are you handling that revelation?" he asked, focusing not on the legal details but on Rachel's internal response.

"Better than I would have expected," she answered truthfully. "I'm concerned, obviously. I'm preparing strategically with my attorney. But I'm not spiraling into panic or getting lost in catastrophic thinking."

A slight smile appeared on Dr. Hughes' face—not amusement but professional satisfaction at observing the practical application of their work together.

"That's significant," he noted. "Not because stress wouldn't be a natural response to this situation, but because you're maintaining function despite legitimate pressure. That's precisely the goal of cortisol fasting."

🔬 He sketched a simple diagram showing stress response over time.

> "Most people approach high-pressure situations in one of two ways," he explained. "Either they suppress stress entirely—denying its existence until it inevitably breaks through in destructive ways—or they surrender to it completely, remaining in a state of heightened activation that eventually leads to burnout."

He tapped the paper between these two extremes. "Cortisol fasting offers a third approach: strategic stress cycling. This isn't about eliminating stress—it's about controlling when it's active and when it's not, preventing the chronic elevation that damages systems while still allowing appropriate activation when needed."

Rachel studied the diagram with interest. "Like interval training for the nervous system?"

"Precisely," Dr. Hughes confirmed.

> "Just as athletes use controlled periods of intensity followed by recovery to strengthen physical systems, you can use deliberate stress cycling to build neurological resilience."

He outlined a comprehensive protocol specifically designed for extended high-stakes situations like custody proceedings:

> **Phase 1: The Strategic Cortisol Window**
> "Most people make the mistake of remaining in stress mode 24/7 during crises," he explained. "They think constant vigilance improves outcomes, when actually it deteriorates decision-making while depleting the very resources needed for effective response."

Instead, Rachel would designate specific hours—perhaps one hour each morning and one hour each evening—for focusing on the custody situation. Outside those windows, she would implement deliberate cortisol reduction techniques to maintain equilibrium.

- ☑ This meant setting clear boundaries around when she would read legal documents, discuss strategy with her attorney, or think about the case. Beyond those designated times, she would intentionally engage in activities that promoted recovery and restoration.

> **Phase 2: The Precision Stress Cycle**
> "The key principle is that stress must always be followed by recovery," he emphasized. "This prevents the chronic elevation that damages systems while still allowing you to engage with legitimate challenges."

Practically, this meant that every time Rachel handled legal tasks or processed difficult emotions related to the custody situation, she would follow with specific recovery practices—breathwork, cold exposure, gentle movement, or meditation—to reset her baseline functioning.

- ☑ She would implement structured transitions between stress engagement and recovery—perhaps five minutes of controlled breathing after legal consultations, or a brief walk outside after reviewing case documents.

> **Phase 3: The Stress-Resilience Threshold**
> "Too little stress creates complacency and lack of motivation," Dr. Hughes explained. "Too much creates panic and impaired thinking. Your goal is to maintain the middle ground—what scientists call 'optimal arousal'—where you're appropriately engaged without becoming overwhelmed."

For this phase, Rachel would implement daily tracking of her stress levels, using both subjective assessment and objective measurements like morning heart rate variability to ensure she remained within the performance zone rather than drifting into either complacency or overwhelm.

- ☑ This meant a consistent morning check-in to assess her baseline stress level, followed by strategic adjustments to her day based on that reading—more recovery if stress was elevated, more engagement if it was unusually low.

"This isn't about avoiding stress," Dr. Hughes concluded. "It's about using it strategically—activating it when its energy serves you and deactivating it when it doesn't. That's how you maintain effectiveness in high-stakes situations without burning yourself out in the process."

Rachel considered the approach thoughtfully. "So I'm not trying to eliminate stress during this custody battle. I'm trying to control it—to use it as a tool rather than being used by it."

> 💡 "Exactly. Most people let stress control them. High performers learn to control stress—activating it intentionally when needed and deactivating it when it's not."

This wasn't about avoiding the fight. It was about fighting effectively—using stress as a strategic resource rather than being consumed by it.

The First Attack: Michael's Psychological Warfare

Rachel was reviewing documents for a client presentation when the email arrived. The notification appeared innocuously in the corner of her screen, but the subject line instantly redirected her attention:

Subject: *Rachel's Parenting History (Case #2023-FC-0478)*

With deliberate intention, she took three deep breaths before opening the message.

The attached document was labeled "Incident Summary for Court Consideration." Its contents represented a methodical catalog of every parenting failure Rachel had committed over the past five years—presented in clinical, dispassionate language that somehow made each item more damning than emotional accusations would have been.

January 12, 2021: Respondent missed child's annual doctor appointment after confirming attendance, requiring rescheduling and disruption to child's routine.

March 4, 2021: Respondent observed checking phone repeatedly during school music performance, child visibly distressed by lack of attention.

June 17, 2021: Respondent arrived 47 minutes late for scheduled pickup without prior notification, leaving child waiting alone after extracurricular activity concluded.

Her pulse quickened as she scrolled through the document, an uncomfortable heat rising in her face. These weren't exaggerations or misrepresentations. They were accurate accounts of her genuine failures—moments when she had prioritized work over her son, when her stress addiction had stolen presence that should have belonged to him.

The email itself contained only a brief message:

For your review prior to our preliminary hearing. We believe this establishes a clear pattern of parental neglect and prioritization of work over the minor child's well-being.

Rachel recognized the tactic immediately. This wasn't just evidence gathering—it was psychological warfare. Michael's lawyer had sent this outside formal channels for a specific purpose: to destabilize her emotionally before their first court appearance, to trigger exactly the stress response that had characterized her previous functioning.

The strategy was elegant in its simplicity. By confronting her with comprehensive documentation of her past failures, they hoped to activate shame, guilt, and defensive reactivity—emotional states that would undermine her current stability and potentially drive her back into visible stress patterns that would support their case.

Six months ago, this approach would have worked perfectly. She would have spiraled into self-recrimination, defensive justification, and panic—likely responding with an emotional message that could later be used against her, or making reactive decisions that compromised her position.

Today, she recognized the trap for what it was.

Taking another deep breath, Rachel moved her cursor away from the reply button. Instead, she saved the document to her legal folder without responding, then closed her email entirely.

The physiological activation remained—her heart still beating faster than normal, a slight tremor in her hands, the warm flush of adrenaline under her skin. But these sensations no longer dictated her actions. She observed them with curious detachment rather than being controlled by them.

The Stress Override Protocol: Shutting Down Emotional Hijacking

Rachel refused to be manipulated. She was in control now. Not Michael. Not her past. Not stress.

She activated the Stress Override Protocol immediately.

Step 1: Acknowledge the Emotion Without Reacting
- ☑ She didn't respond to the email. She didn't argue in her head. She wrote one sentence in her notebook:

💬 *"My past mistakes do not define me."*

Step 2: Physically Release the Stress Surge
- ☑ She went straight into a 5-minute breathwork session—a technique Dr. Hughes had taught her specifically for moments when emotions threatened to override logical thinking.
- ☑ *Inhale for 4 seconds → Hold for 7 seconds → Exhale for 8 seconds.*
- ☑ Within minutes, her heart rate dropped, the trembling in her hands subsided, and the heat in her face began to cool. The physical reset was breaking the escalation cycle before it could fully develop.

> **Step 3: Reframe the Attack as an Opportunity**
> ☑ Instead of seeing this as a personal attack, she reframed it:
>
> 💬 *"This is not an attack. This is my chance to prove who I am now."*

The shift was subtle but powerful. Rather than viewing Michael's evidence as a threat to be defended against, she recognized it as an opportunity to demonstrate the contrast between who she had been and who she had become.

Michael wanted her to break. She wasn't going to give him the satisfaction. She was playing the long game now.

The Turning Point: Rachel Fires Back—With Strategy, Not Emotion

Later that night, Rachel met with her lawyer, Catherine Reyes, in the attorney's downtown office.

Catherine expected her to be emotional, defensive, and scattered—the typical state of clients facing custody challenges, especially when confronted with documented evidence of past parenting failures.

Instead, she was calm. Focused. Ready.

"We're not going to play his game," Rachel said firmly, spreading her organized notes across Catherine's desk. "We're going to prove, without a doubt, that **I am the mother I say I am now**."

Instead of reacting to Michael's accusations, they built a case that focused on who Rachel was today:

- ☑ **Evidence of how she had changed.** Therapeutic records documenting her recovery from burnout. Weekly schedules showing her consistent presence in Ethan's life over recent months. Her transformed work arrangement at Vertex that prioritized parenting responsibilities.

- ☑ Character references from Emily, colleagues, and especially Dr. Hughes, whose professional assessment of her transformation would carry particular weight with the court.
- ☑ A structured parenting plan showing her emotional and logistical stability—detailing how she had rebuilt her life specifically to be more available and present for Ethan.

Catherine nodded approvingly as they developed their strategy. "Most clients want to attack their ex or deny evidence. You're doing something smarter—acknowledging the past while proving it's no longer relevant."

Michael wanted her to crumble under stress.

Rachel was about to show him just how unshakable she had become.

The Attack She Didn't See Coming

A week later, Rachel walked into Catherine's office, expecting to discuss parenting plans.

Catherine slid a new document across the desk.

Subject: Psychological Fitness for Parenting Evaluation

Her stomach dropped.

Michael wasn't just attacking her ability to parent. He was claiming she was mentally unfit to raise their son.

Rachel scanned the accusations:

"History of chronic anxiety and stress mismanagement."
"Documented periods of emotional instability."
"Failed relationships due to workaholism and detachment."

Every therapy session she had ever attended, every moment of burnout, every breakdown—Michael had found a way to use it against her, framing her recovery journey not as evidence of growth but as proof of inherent instability.

And the worst part? It wasn't a lie.

Michael wasn't making anything up—he was just framing it in a way that made her look unfit, using her efforts to heal as evidence that she was fundamentally broken.

She had spent years fixing herself. She had rebuilt her entire life. She had proven—at least to herself—that she was stronger now.

But what if the court didn't see it that way?

Why Stress Makes You Question Everything (Even When You've Changed)

🔬 Dr. Hughes had warned her that stress can trigger old neural pathways—bringing back emotions and doubts that no longer serve you.

Here's why high-stakes stress makes people doubt themselves:

1. The Brain Defaults to Old Thought Patterns
Under extreme stress, the brain reactivates old survival mechanisms. Rachel's mind instantly replayed every failure, every panic attack, every moment she had broken under pressure.

☑ Even though she had healed, her brain was telling her she hadn't. The neural pathways formed during years of stress addiction were still physically present, ready to be reactivated when similar threat conditions appeared.

2. The "What If They're Right?" Effect
When an old weakness is thrown in your face, it's hard not to question your growth. Rachel had worked so hard to change, but now she wondered if it was enough. Was Michael right? Was she fundamentally unstable?

☑ High-pressure situations force people to prove to themselves that they've changed. The doubt isn't just external—it becomes an internal questioning that can undermine even the most solid transformation if not recognized and addressed.

3. The Fight-or-Flight Hijack
When the body senses a threat (losing custody of her son), cortisol skyrockets. Logic shuts down. Only fear and survival instincts remain. The prefrontal cortex—responsible for rational thinking and perspective—becomes less active, while the amygdala—the brain's threat detection center—takes control.

☑ Stress pushes people to react emotionally instead of strategically. This is why high-stakes situations often bring out the worst in people, even when they've done significant personal growth work.

Michael wasn't just testing Rachel's parenting—he was testing whether she truly owned her new identity.

Would she revert to her old patterns or stay in control?

Step 1: The Preemptive Cortisol Detox

Rachel knew if she let stress hijack her now, she would lose everything.

She had two choices:
- Let fear take over and react emotionally.
- Use cortisol fasting to override her fight-or-flight response and stay in control.

She chose the second option.

The Preemptive Cortisol Detox: Stopping the Spiral Before It Start

1. **Instant Physiological Reset**
   - ☑ She left the office, put on her running shoes, and sprinted until her lungs burned, pushing her body to the physical limit.

Why? Intense movement forces cortisol to be processed out of the bloodstream faster. Exercise triggers the release of endorphins and BDNF (Brain-Derived Neurotrophic Factor), both of which help regulate emotional responses and improve cognitive function. The physical exertion creates a legitimate outlet for the fight-or-flight energy that would otherwise remain trapped in her system.

2. **Controlled Emotional Reprocessing**
   - ☑ Instead of suppressing emotions, she gave herself 15 minutes to feel everything—setting a timer and allowing all the fear, anger, and hurt to surface without judgment.

Why? Studies show that setting a time limit on emotional reactions helps the brain regulate them faster. Suppressed emotions intensify and persist, while acknowledged emotions can be processed and released. The time boundary prevents wallowing while still allowing necessary emotional processing.

3. **Prefrontal Cortex Activation (The Logical Override)**
   - ☑ She sat down and wrote:

> *"What would a rational person do next? Not emotional—rational."*

Why? Engaging the logical brain pulls the body out of panic mode. Writing activates the prefrontal cortex, which stress hormones typically suppress. By deliberately engaging this area through structured analytical thinking, she was counteracting the amygdala's dominance in the stress response.

Stress wasn't going to break her this time. She had trained for this.

Step 2: Controlling the Narrative—Before Michael Could

Rachel met with Catherine the next morning.

Her lawyer expected her to be defensive. Emotional. Scattered.

Instead, she was calm. Prepared. Unshakable.

"We're not reacting to Michael," Rachel stated, spreading out her organized notes. "We're controlling the narrative."

They built their strategy:

1. **Own the Past, But Prove the Growth**
   - ☑ Instead of denying her past struggles, Rachel leaned into them.
   - ☑ She provided documented proof of her transformation—therapy records, professional assessments, and witness statements.

   💬 *"Yes, I struggled. And here's everything I've done to ensure my son has a stable, healthy mother today."*

   Rather than allowing Michael to use her past against her, she would reframe it as evidence of her commitment to growth and healing, specifically for Ethan's benefit.

2. **Shift the Focus to Michael's Motivations**
   - ☑ They gathered evidence that Michael's lawsuit wasn't about their son's well-being—it was about control.

   💬 *"Why is he doing this now? And why does he suddenly think I'm unfit only after I've rebuilt my life?"*

   Catherine would investigate the timing of the petition—coming only after Rachel had genuinely transformed—to suggest this was about power rather than protection.

3. Flip the Psychological Fitness Test Against Him
☑ Michael had opened the door for a psychological review—so Rachel's team counter-filed to have him evaluated, too.

💬 *"If my past struggles are relevant, then let's take a full look at both parents' mental health history."*

By requesting both parents undergo the same evaluation, they would level the playing field while showing Rachel had nothing to hide.

Michael thought she would collapse under the weight of her past.

Instead, she had turned his attack into her greatest advantage.

The Courtroom Showdown: Can She Stay in Control?

The courtroom was cold and sterile.

Michael sat across from her, smug, confident. His lawyer had a stack of papers in front of him—evidence of her past failures. The judge was stone-faced, unreadable.

This was real. This was happening. And she had one shot to prove she had changed.

Then, Michael's lawyer stood up. And he went straight for the kill.

"Your Honor, I'd like to read an email from Ms. Summers to her former employer, dated two years ago."

Rachel's breath hitched.

Rachel's Own Words (From Two Years Ago): *"I can't do this anymore. I feel like I'm drowning. I'm completely overwhelmed, and I don't even have time to be a mother. Something has to give, and it can't be Ethan. I need help."*

The courtroom was silent.

Michael's lawyer let the words settle. Let them sting.

This was the moment Michael had been waiting for.

Because no matter how much she had changed, no matter how much she had improved—this was still who she used to be.

And now, she had to prove she wasn't that woman anymore.

The 10-Second Cortisol Reset

Rachel didn't have time for a long meditation or a cold shower.

She needed a way to shut down stress—instantly.

So she used the 10-Second Cortisol Reset, a neuroscience-backed method to override the stress response in real-time.

1. **Slow Down the Heart Rate**
   💡 The fastest way to stop stress is to slow the breath.

   ☑ She inhaled deeply for 4 seconds—held for 7—exhaled for 8.
   ☑ Within seconds, her heart rate dropped. The cardiac rhythm shift triggered what scientists call "respiratory sinus arrhythmia"—a physiological state that signals safety to the nervous system.

2. **Reframe the Threat**
   💡 The brain only panics when it sees something as dangerous.

   ☑ She reminded herself:
   💬 "This is not an attack. This is an opportunity to prove who I am."

   This cognitive reframing changed how her brain processed the situation—from threat to challenge, from danger to opportunity.

> **3. Activate the Logical Brain**
> 💡 Emotional reactions lose cases. Rational responses win them.
>
> ☑ She asked herself:
> 💬 *"What would a calm, confident person say right now?"*
>
> This question shifted brain activity from the amygdala (emotional center) to the prefrontal cortex (logical center), allowing her to respond strategically rather than reactively.

The stress was still there—but it was no longer in control.

The Perfect Response That Changed Everything

Rachel turned to the judge, voice steady.

"Your Honor, I don't deny that I wrote that email. And I don't deny that two years ago, I was struggling."

She didn't fight the accusation. She owned it.

Michael's lawyer had expected her to crumble. Instead, she leaned into the fire. "But that email isn't a reflection of who I am today. It's proof of how far I've come."

The courtroom shifted. Michael's lawyer blinked, thrown off balance.

Rachel wasn't defending her past—she was proving her transformation.

Her lawyer handed over a folder.

Inside?

Therapist evaluations proving her emotional stability. Character references from Emily, her employer, and even Ethan's teachers. Parenting schedules showing she had been fully present for the last several months. A comprehensive assessment from Dr. Hughes documenting her recovery from burnout and the systems she had built to prevent its return.

"I don't expect this court to judge me on who I used to be," Rachel said, her voice growing stronger. "I expect it to judge me on who I am now—the mother who recognized her failings and did everything humanly possible to become the parent her son deserves."

Michael had tried to use her past to define her. But Rachel had turned it into proof of her evolution.

This wasn't just about custody anymore. This was about Rachel reclaiming her entire narrative.

The Verdict That Changed Everything
Rachel sat in her apartment, staring at her phone.

The judge's decision was coming today.

Everything she had fought for, every piece of growth, every battle—it all came down to this.

Would she get to keep shared custody of Ethan, or would Michael win?

She had done everything right. She had stayed in control, proven her growth, and fought back strategically.

But none of it mattered if the judge didn't see what she saw in herself.

The phone rang.

"Rachel, I have the ruling," Catherine said. "You're going to want to sit down."

Her stomach twisted. She braced for the worst.

"The court ruled in favor of maintaining shared custody. Michael's petition for full custody was denied."

Rachel's breath caught. She had won.

Michael didn't get what he wanted. The court had ruled that Rachel was a fit mother—that her transformation was real and substantial enough to matter.

But before she could celebrate, the next words hit her like a punch to the gut.

"But... there's a condition."

The Condition That Shook Her to the Core

Rachel gripped the phone.

"The court is requiring a 90-day psychological evaluation and co-parenting supervision."

Her stomach dropped.

Even though she had won custody, the court still didn't fully trust her. She had to prove herself. Again.

For 90 days, every interaction with her son would be monitored, every decision scrutinized, and her parenting evaluated by professionals, looking for any sign that she might revert to her old patterns.

It wasn't a loss. But it sure as hell didn't feel like a win.

Her hands tightened into fists.

She had changed. She knew that.

But the world still saw her as the woman she used to be.

And now, she had to prove her worth all over again.

Why Stress Triggers Resentment— and How to Stop It

Rachel felt something rising in her chest—something dark, heavy.

Resentment.

She had done the work. She had rebuilt her life. She had faced her demons and emerged stronger. And still, she had to prove herself?

🔬 Dr. Hughes had explained that stress often leads to resentment—because it makes people feel powerless.

Why Stress Makes People Resentful:
1. It Makes You Feel Like Your Effort Isn't Enough
Rachel had changed, but she was still being judged for her past.

When you put in the work and people don't believe it, stress turns into bitterness. The brain interprets this as injustice, triggering a cascade of negative emotions that can undermine even the most significant progress.

2. It Traps You in a Cycle of "Why Me?" Thinking
Stress triggers comparison and injustice thinking.

💬 *"Why do I have to prove myself when Michael never had to?"*

This thought pattern activates regions of the brain associated with perceived unfairness, creating a negative spiral that can be difficult to escape.

3. It Makes You Want to Give Up
Resentment is mental exhaustion—it makes people feel like nothing will ever be good enough.

That's how stress wins—by making you think the fight isn't worth it. By draining your motivation and making continued effort seem pointless.

Rachel wasn't going to let stress turn into resentment.

She had come too far for that.

Step 1: Releasing the Need for Instant Validation
Rachel stared out the window, feeling the frustration coil inside her.

She had been waiting for the world to recognize her growth.

She had expected a moment when everything just clicked—where the judge would see her transformation and acknowledge it completely, where her value as a mother would be unquestionably affirmed.

But that's not how change works.

Growth doesn't happen in a courtroom. It happens in the everyday moments no one sees. It happens in the small decisions, the consistent choices, the private victories that accumulate into genuine transformation.

She wasn't proving herself for Michael, for the judge, or for anyone else. She was proving herself for her son.

And that would take more than a court ruling—it would take time.

Step 2: Turning the 90-Day Condition Into an Advantage
Rachel called her lawyer back.

"This 90-day condition—how closely will I be monitored?"

"It means Michael has a say in co-parenting decisions, and there will be scheduled check-ins with a family therapist. It's meant to be a transition period, not a punishment."

Rachel exhaled slowly.

So it wasn't a restriction—it was an opportunity.

This wasn't a test she had to pass. It was a chance to prove, day by day, that she was the mother she had fought to become.

Instead of resisting it, she was going to use it.

The 90 days would become her showcase—each interaction with Ethan, each parenting decision, each co-parenting exchange with Michael would demonstrate the reality of her transformation.
She would turn what was intended as scrutiny into a platform for proving exactly who she had become.

Step 3: The "Long Game" Stress Strategy
Rachel knew she had to shift her mindset.
This wasn't about winning or losing. This was about playing the long game.

She had to train her nervous system for long-term resilience—not just short-term victories.

The Long Game Stress Strategy:

1. **Stop Seeking Instant Wins**
   💡 Stress comes from needing immediate results. Growth doesn't work that way.

   ☑ She reminded herself daily:
   💬 *"This isn't about proving myself today. It's about showing up consistently."*

Each day was simply another opportunity to demonstrate who she had become—not a pass/fail test, but one small piece of a larger pattern.

2. **Use Stress as a Daily Compass, Not a Threat**
   💡 Instead of fearing stress, use it as feedback.

   ☑ She tracked her emotions every night:
   💬 *"Did I stay present with Ethan today?"*
   💬 *"Did I let resentment creep in?"*
   💬 *"Did I handle today better than I would have a year ago?"*

These questions transformed her relationship with stress—from something to fear into data that could guide her continued growth.

3. **Keep the Big Picture in Mind**
   💡 The goal wasn't just to survive 90 days—it was to build a lifelong bond with her son.

> She told herself
> 💬 *"This doesn't end in 90 days. This is forever."*

This wasn't a restriction—it was the first chapter in the rest of her life.

The Moment Everything Changed

One week later, Rachel picked up Ethan for their scheduled visit.

For the first time since the court battle, he looked at her differently.

"Mom, are you okay?" he asked as they walked toward her car, his voice carrying genuine concern.

Rachel blinked.

Ethan had always known her as the stressed-out, distracted, overworked mother.

He had always seen the exhaustion in her eyes, the tension in her shoulders, the divided attention that meant she was never fully present even when physically there.

But now? He saw something else.

He saw peace. He saw confidence. He saw presence.

Despite the court battle, despite the 90-day condition, despite everything Michael had thrown at her—she wasn't stressed. She wasn't fragmented. She wasn't falling apart.

She was calmer and more present than ever.

Rachel smiled, resting her hand gently on his shoulder. "I'm better than okay. I'm here."

His tentative smile in response told her everything she needed to know. The custody battle, the court's conditions, Michael's attacks—none of it mattered compared to this moment of genuine connection with her son.

This was what she had been fighting for all along.

The Final Test: Can She Prove It?
Throughout the 90-day evaluation period, Rachel maintained her cortisol fasting protocol rigorously.

> ☑ She kept her scheduled "stress windows" for dealing with legal matters, containing the emotional impact of the case to specific times rather than allowing it to bleed into her entire life.
> ☑ She followed every stressful interaction—whether with Michael, the court-appointed therapist, or her attorney—with deliberate recovery practices that reset her nervous system to baseline.
> ☑ She tracked her stress levels daily, making strategic adjustments to maintain optimal functioning rather than drifting into either complacency or overwhelm.

The results were undeniable:
She remained calm during co-parenting exchanges that once would have triggered defensive reactions.

She stayed present with Ethan during their time together, rather than being mentally preoccupied with the case.

She approached the therapy sessions as opportunities to demonstrate her growth rather than threats to be managed.

Most significantly, she didn't just survive the 90-day evaluation—she thrived during it, showing a level of stability, presence, and emotional regulation that surprised even those who knew her best.

The final evaluation from the court-appointed therapist stated it plainly: "Ms. Summers has demonstrated consistent emotional stability, appropriate parenting skills, and a genuine commitment to her son's well-being. The transformation in her functioning appears substantial and sustainable."

When the 90 days ended and the supervision was lifted, the victory felt complete in a way the court ruling alone had not.

She hadn't just won legally—she had proven, through consistent daily choices, that her transformation was real.

What Comes Next? When You've Mastered Stress, But The World Still Runs On It

Rachel had won her custody battle by controlling her cortisol, applying strategic stress fasting, and remaining present even under extreme pressure. She had reconnected with her son and was rebuilding their relationship one day at a time.

But as she looked around at her workplace, at the social pressures, at the constant digital stress triggers that surrounded her daily, she realized her journey wasn't complete:

> 💬 *How do I maintain this balance when the entire world seems built to keep people stressed and exhausted?*

She had mastered her internal response to stress, but the external environment remained unchanged—a world designed to keep cortisol chronically elevated, attention perpetually fragmented, and energy continuously depleted.

She was beginning to understand that personal mastery was just the first step. The deeper challenge was creating systems that could reset her entire relationship with cortisol—permanently rewiring her body's stress response even in a world designed to keep it triggered.

Dr. Hughes had helped her understand that this wasn't just a personal health issue but a broader cultural challenge—one that affected millions of high-performers trapped in cycles of stress addiction without recognizing the patterns destroying their health, relationships, and true potential.

As Rachel watched her colleagues at Vertex continue to operate in the same burnout patterns she had escaped, she wondered if there might be a way to share what she had learned—to help others recognize and break free from the cortisol cycles keeping them perpetually exhausted yet unable to stop.

And discovering how to achieve that complete cortisol reset—not just for herself but potentially for others—would be her next challenge.

CHAPTER 9: THE CORTISOL MASTERY BLUEPRINT

Mastery Over Cortisol—How to Turn Your Greatest Enemy Into Your Superpower

When Everything Falls Apart at Once

Rachel's phone vibrated against the polished surface of her desk. Michael's name flashed on the screen. Her ex-husband rarely called during work hours—an unspoken agreement they'd established after the divorce.

Something was wrong.

"Michael? What's—"

"Rachel—" His voice was tight with barely controlled panic. "It's Ethan. We're in an ambulance headed to Memorial. He—" A shaky breath. "He had some kind of severe allergic reaction at school. It's bad."

The world stopped.

Her son. Emergency. Hospital. The words collided in her brain like shrapnel.

In an instant, every system in her body prepared to do what it had been evolutionarily programmed to do: flood with stress hormones, activate emergency response, enter survival mode. This wasn't a difficult client or a tight deadline. This was primal. Visceral. The ultimate trigger.

As she grabbed her keys, a single thought surfaced through the rising tide of panic: If there was ever a situation where stress was not just expected but appropriate—where the cortisol flood seemed not just inevitable but necessary—this was it.

She fumbled with her phone, hitting Dr. Hughes' number on speed dial as she raced to her car.

As she pulled away from Vertex's parking lot, Rachel felt something unprecedented happening in her body—a stress response so powerful it seemed to create its own gravitational pull, threatening to collapse her hard-won recovery into a singularity of panic.

💬 *If I can't maintain control now, I never will.*

Dr. Hughes answered on the second ring, his voice instantly grounding as Rachel explained the situation. He guided her through immediate stabilization techniques as she navigated traffic toward the hospital, promising to talk her through something more advanced once she arrived.

The Perfect Storm of Triggers

Rachel pushed through the emergency room doors, scanning for Michael.

She spotted him by the nurses' station, pacing with his phone pressed to his ear. His face was drawn with worry, but there was something else in his expression—a softness that seemed out of place amid the crisis.

"I know, I know," he was saying, his voice low and intimate. "I'll call you when we know more.

Yes... I miss you too."

Rachel slowed her approach, something in his tone triggering a warning flare in her mind.

He saw her and quickly ended the call. "Rachel—thank God. They've taken him back for assessment."

"Who was that?" The question emerged before she'd consciously formed it.

Michael's expression shifted—guilt flashing briefly before he recovered. "Just... checking in with work."

His phone vibrated in his hand. And in that moment—the universe's cruel sense of timing on full display—the screen lit up with an incoming call.

Emily's name and photo clear on the display.

Michael fumbled to silence it, but the damage was done. Their eyes met, and in that single moment, everything crystallized.

The realization hit Rachel like a physical blow. Emily—her best friend, who had supported her through her burnout recovery, who knew intimately what Michael had put her through during their divorce, who was godmother to Ethan—was having an affair with her ex-husband.

In any other circumstance, this betrayal alone would have been enough to send her stress response skyrocketing. Combined with Ethan's medical emergency, it created the perfect neurological storm.

Rachel could actually feel each system activating—her amygdala firing, cortisol flooding her bloodstream, her heart rate accelerating, her muscles tensing for fight-or-flight.

Before Rachel could respond, the emergency doors opened again, and Emily rushed in, breathless as though she'd been running. She froze when she saw them both standing there.

"Oh—you're here already," she said to Rachel, her expression shifting from surprise to something more complex—guilt mingled with determination. "They're... still assessing Ethan?"

The question directed at Michael, not Rachel, was the final confirmation. The sheer audacity of their pretense—acting as though they hadn't betrayed her in the most fundamental way—created a third layer of threat response on top of the existing crisis.

Michael had the decency to look ashamed as his gaze shifted between the two women. "Emily called when she heard about Ethan," he explained weakly.

Dr. Hughes' words from their phone conversation echoed in Rachel's mind: "This isn't a setback, Rachel. It's an opportunity for the most advanced protocol—the one I've been waiting to share until you were ready."

Rachel took a measured breath, feeling the familiar techniques she'd mastered over months of recovery slide into place. But something told her they wouldn't be enough—not for this, not for what felt like the perfect convergence of every possible trigger—a medical emergency with her son and the sudden discovery of the ultimate betrayal by the two people she had trusted most.

A doctor approached, clipboard in hand. "Ms. Summers? I'm Dr. Patel. Your son is stabilizing, but we need some information about potential allergies."

As Michael moved closer, his face a mask of parental concern that betrayed nothing of his betrayal, Rachel realized she was facing a test unlike any other.

If she could maintain control now—in this perfect storm of medical emergency, personal betrayal, and professional demands—she could maintain it anywhere, anytime.

But how?

Beyond Recovery: The Neurological Timeline Intervention

🔬 Dr. Hughes had explained it quickly during their brief call as she'd driven to the hospital—a protocol so advanced he hadn't shared it until now. Until she was ready. Until she faced a trigger powerful enough to necessitate it.

"What you're experiencing isn't just about Ethan's current situation," he had said, his voice calm through the phone. "Your brain is activating every stored memory of threat, every encoded fear about your child, and projecting catastrophic futures—all simultaneously."

"This isn't the time for stress management, " Rachel had whispered, her voice tight. "My son is—"

"This is exactly the time," he had interrupted gently. "Because we're not going to manage this stress. We're going to use it to rewrite your entire neurological relationship with threat."

> He had explained rapidly: The most revolutionary discovery in neuroscience wasn't just that the brain could change—but that it was most malleable during states of intense activation. The very moment when stress was at its peak was precisely when the neural networks were most receptive to permanent recoding.

> "What you've been doing until now has been rewiring your present response to stress," he had said. "What we're about to do is rewrite your brain's entire relationship with threat—past, present, and future simultaneously."

This wasn't stress management. This wasn't even stress immunity.

This was neurological time travel.

Now, standing in the hospital corridor with Dr. Patel asking questions, Michael hovering nearby, and Emily's presence a constant reminder of betrayal, Rachel initiated the protocol Dr. Hughes had outlined.

Phase 1: Neural Inventory Mapping

As the doctor explained Ethan's condition—anaphylaxis from an unknown allergen, still being stabilized—Rachel initiated the first phase of the protocol.

Neural Inventory Mapping.

With practiced precision, she began identifying each activated threat network: the primal parental fear for her child; the fresh wound of betrayal from Emily; the complex history with Michael; the professional habit of maintaining control in crisis.

Each neural pathway lit up in her awareness like circuits on a motherboard.

> 🔔 This wasn't metaphorical. Research had shown that bringing conscious awareness to specific neural networks actually altered their function. By precisely identifying each activated threat system rather than experiencing them as an undifferentiated mass of panic, she was already beginning to reshape her brain's response.

"Has Ethan ever had allergic reactions before?" Dr. Patel asked.

"Minor ones to certain laundry detergents," Rachel replied, her voice steadier than she expected. "Nothing food-related that we've identified."

Michael was adding something about what Ethan had eaten at lunch. Emily stood slightly apart now, her eyes darting between Rachel and Michael.

The mapping continued, Rachel's awareness expanding to include not just primary threats but the complex patterns connecting them—how her history with Michael amplified her fear for Ethan, how Emily's betrayal intensified her sense of isolation in crisis, how all of these fed into her deeper patterns of cortisol addiction.

For the first time, she wasn't just experiencing these responses—she was observing their complete neural architecture.

The Brain's Emergency Response System

As Rachel deepened the mapping process, she became aware of how her brain's alarm system was constructed. Dr. Hughes had taught her that this wasn't just psychological awareness—it was actual neurobiological change occurring in real time.

> When faced with multiple threats, most people experience them as a single overwhelming emotional tsunami. But by mapping each distinct threat network, Rachel was activating a critical brain region called the prefrontal cortex—the part responsible for rational thinking that typically goes offline during stress.
>
> The parental fear for Ethan registered as activity in her brain's most primitive regions—the instinctual protective circuits that have kept children safe since humans first walked the earth. The betrayal by Emily and Michael activated the social pain networks, the same brain regions that process physical pain. The need to maintain control in crisis engaged her identity centers, the neural networks that defined who she was and how she responded to the world.

By specifically naming and locating each threat response in her awareness, Rachel was doing something remarkable—she was keeping her thinking brain online during a crisis that would normally shut it down entirely. This wasn't about denying emotions; it was about experiencing them with her complete brain rather than just the reactive parts.

Dr. Patel continued asking detailed questions about Ethan's medical history. Despite the emotional complexity of the situation, Rachel found herself able to provide clear, comprehensive information—a direct result of keeping her cognitive systems functioning alongside her emotional responses.

"You're remarkably composed," Dr. Patel noted with professional appreciation. "That's incredibly helpful right now."

Rachel nodded slightly. What the doctor couldn't know was that this composure wasn't the result of emotional suppression—quite the opposite. She was experiencing all the appropriate emotions, but without the neurological chaos that typically accompanied them.

The Neural Inventory Mapping continued creating a crucial foundation for what came next—the even more advanced phases of the protocol that would permanently transform her brain's relationship with threat.

Phase 2: Timeline Decompression

Rachel moved into the second phase—Timeline Decompression.

> 🔬 Dr. Hughes had explained that stress responses collapse time: past traumas, present threats, and anticipated future disasters become neurologically indistinguishable. The brain processes them as a single overwhelming now, creating a cortisol response proportional to their combined weight rather than the present reality.

Timeline Decompression reversed this process.

> With extraordinary clarity, she separated the neural pathways encoding past threats from present reality: her history with Michael was distinct from this current emergency; Emily's betrayal was a separate issue from Ethan's medical condition; her professional identity existed independently from her role as mother.

What would normally have blurred together into an overwhelming emotional tsunami remained distinct, manageable neural networks—each requiring different responses, none requiring emergency cortisol activation.

"We need to know if he has any medications or other health conditions," the doctor was saying, looking between Rachel and Michael.

"No ongoing medications," Rachel replied, her voice steady. "He had bronchitis last winter but has been healthy since."

She was simultaneously processing the medical information, implementing the protocol, and navigating the emotional complexity of standing between her ex-husband and former best friend.

The physical sensations of stress—the tight chest, the shallow breathing, the trembling hands—began shifting as her brain recognized that what it had perceived as a single catastrophic threat was actually several distinct situations, only one of which (Ethan's medical condition) required immediate attention.

And even that wasn't served by cortisol overload.

Separating Past, Present, and Future

> The Timeline Decompression created a remarkable shift in Rachel's perception. Typically, during high stress, the brain's time-processing systems malfunction—past traumas feel as though they're happening again, present challenges feel insurmountable, and future fears feel inevitable.

> 🔔 Dr. Hughes had explained that this happens because stress hormones disrupt the normal functioning of the hippocampus—the brain region that helps place experiences in their proper time context. When the hippocampus is flooded with stress chemicals, everything collapses into a single overwhelming now.

Rachel could actually feel her brain's time-processing systems coming back online as she implemented this phase of the protocol. The divorce with Michael—a painful event from years ago—regained its proper temporal distance. It had happened, she had survived it, and it wasn't happening again right now. Emily's betrayal remained a present issue requiring future attention, but it wasn't life-threatening, despite the social pain it caused. Ethan's medical situation stood alone as the one genuine present emergency, but even that was already showing signs of improvement.

"We've got his vital signs stabilizing," Dr. Patel noted, checking his chart. "The antihistamines are working effectively."

Rachel absorbed this information with a sense of relief that felt physically different from her normal experience. Instead of the temporary emotional spike that usually came with good news during crisis—quickly followed by the search for the next threat—she felt a genuine, sustained reduction in physical tension. Her breathing deepened naturally, her shoulders relaxed away from her ears, her jaw unclenched.

This wasn't just psychological comfort; it was actual neurobiological change—her autonomic nervous system downshifting in response to accurate time perception rather than remaining locked in emergency mode.

As they walked toward the elevator to follow Ethan to his room, Rachel noticed something extraordinary: even with genuine concerns still present, her body wasn't producing the excessive stress hormones that had been her lifelong pattern during crisis. By decompressing the timeline, she had provided her brain with the context it needed to generate appropriate responses rather than emergency overreactions.

The past remained in the past. The future contained multiple possibilities rather than inevitable disasters. The present became navigable rather than overwhelming.

This wasn't denial or emotional suppression. It was the brain's natural functioning when freed from the distortion of collapsed time perception.

Phase 3: Projected Outcome Restructuring

As Rachel moved into the third phase—Projected Outcome Restructuring—something remarkable began happening in her neurological processing.

> 🕯 Dr. Hughes had explained that the stress response largely comes from the brain's anticipation of catastrophic outcomes. But these projections are rarely accurate—they're exaggerated simulations based on past experiences and worst-case scenarios, not objective assessments of likely futures.

The catastrophic futures her brain had automatically generated began reorganizing into evidence-based possibilities:

Ethan was already stabilizing with proper medical treatment—not getting worse as her fear center had projected.

The betrayal would need to be addressed, but not during this emergency—and it wouldn't undo her entire social support system as her threat networks had initially calculated.

Her relationship with Emily was irrevocably changed, but this didn't threaten her survival or even her well-being beyond the immediate emotional pain.

This wasn't denial or suppression. It was neurological efficiency—her brain's threat-response system recalibrating to actual danger levels rather than perceived catastrophes.

"We're moving him to a room upstairs," Dr. Patel explained. "The epinephrine is working, but we want to monitor him overnight to ensure there's no secondary reaction."

Rachel nodded, mentally reorganizing her schedule, calculating when she needed to contact Vertex, planning what she'd need to bring from home for Ethan's overnight stay.

But these thoughts occurred without the frantic edge of stress-based thinking. They flowed with unusual clarity—each consideration distinct, none triggering the cascade of worst-case scenarios that typically accompanied crisis planning.

Emily stepped forward tentatively. "I can go get some things from your apartment if you want to stay with him."

A week ago, Rachel would have accepted the offer gratefully. Now, knowing what she did, a complex emotion surfaced—but importantly, it arose as information rather than activation.

"That won't be necessary," she replied evenly. "Michael can stay while I get what Ethan needs."

She registered Emily's flinch at the subtle boundary, but felt no corresponding surge of either vindication or guilt—just clarity about what was appropriate in this new reality.

Rewiring the Brain's Prediction Machine

As Rachel continued restructuring how her brain projected potential futures, she became aware of what neuroscientists call "the predictive brain"—the mind's constant activity of anticipating what might happen next. Dr. Hughes had explained that the brain is essentially a prediction machine, constantly creating simulations of future possibilities to prepare for them.

> Under stress, this prediction system gets hijacked. Instead of generating a range of realistic possibilities, the brain fixates on worst-case scenarios and assigns them unrealistically high probabilities.

> This evolutionary mechanism once helped our ancestors prepare for genuine threats like predator attacks, but in modern life, it creates unnecessary suffering without improving outcomes.

What Rachel was experiencing wasn't positive thinking or wishful denial—it was teaching her brain's prediction systems to calculate actual probabilities based on evidence rather than fear. The medical facts indicated Ethan was responding well to treatment. The betrayal was painful but not life-threatening. Her work obligations could be rearranged without catastrophic consequences.

As this restructuring deepened, Rachel noticed something fascinating happening in her body. The tight knot in her stomach began to loosen. The tension headache that had been forming at the base of her skull started to dissolve. Her breathing naturally deepened without conscious effort. These weren't just psychological changes but actual physiological responses to her brain's recalibrated threat assessment.

"We'll need to identify the specific allergen," Dr. Patel explained as they walked toward the elevator. Once we know what triggered this reaction, we can develop an appropriate management plan."

Rachel nodded, her mind already processing this information through her restructured prediction system. Instead of catastrophizing about life-threatening allergies lurking everywhere, her brain generated practical considerations: they would need to modify Ethan's diet, inform his school, and possibly carry emergency medication. These were manageable challenges, not existential threats.

This restructuring created what psychologists call "cognitive flexibility"—the ability to adapt thinking based on changing circumstances rather than remaining locked in rigid threat patterns. As Rachel stepped into the elevator with Michael, Emily hovering uncertainly nearby, she experienced this flexibility in real time—her mind generating adaptive responses to a complex situation rather than reactive panic.

"Fourth floor," the nurse mentioned as she pressed the button. "The pediatric unit has private rooms for parents to stay overnight."

This practical information registered without triggering the stress cascade that would typically accompany thoughts of hospital stays. Rachel's restructured projection system recognized this as helpful information rather than another threatening development.

That was the key difference—her brain was processing reality more accurately rather than filtering everything through fear-based distortion.

Phase 4: Memory Reconsolidation Targeting

As they followed Ethan's gurney to the elevator, Rachel initiated the fourth phase—perhaps the most revolutionary aspect of the protocol.

Memory Reconsolidation Targeting.

> According to the latest neuroscience, memories aren't static recordings but active reconstructions that become temporarily malleable when accessed. This process—reconsolidation—creates a brief window when memories can be permanently altered before being restored.
>
> By accessing stress-related memories during an active stress state while simultaneously maintaining her cortisol levels in check, Rachel was effectively rewriting how those memories would be stored and accessed in the future.

As the elevator doors closed, with Michael and Emily awkwardly positioned at opposite corners, Rachel deliberately brought to mind key stress memories:

The day Michael had announced he wanted a divorce, leaving her with three-year-old Ethan and a mortgage she could barely afford.

The previous time Ethan had been hospitalized with a high fever, she'd sat alone in a similar corridor feeling completely overwhelmed.

The moment she'd first recognized her burnout, standing in her bathroom unable to remember if she'd already shampooed her hair.

But instead of experiencing these memories with their original emotional signatures, she remained in her current state of controlled clarity—effectively creating a neurological mismatch that forced her brain to update how these events were encoded.

She wasn't just managing stress better in the present moment. She was literally rewriting how her brain had stored stress experiences from her past—altering their emotional content and weakening their power as triggers.

It wasn't that the memories changed—the events remained the same. But their neurological impact, their power to activate stress pathways, was being permanently diminished.

"He'll be in Room 412," a nurse informed them as the elevator reached the fourth floor. "Only two visitors at a time please."

Rachel turned to Michael and Emily. "You two take the first shift. I'll get his things from home."

The look that passed between them—guilt, relief, confusion—registered in Rachel's awareness without triggering an emotional response. She was operating from a place beyond reactivity—not through effortful restraint, but through fundamental neurological reorganization.

Rewriting Emotional Memory

What Rachel experienced during the Memory Reconsolidation phase wasn't just psychological reframing—it was an actual biological process changing how her brain stored emotional experiences.

> Dr. Hughes had explained that memories aren't static recordings like computer files but active processes that get rebuilt each time we recall them. When we access a memory, the brain briefly places it in an unstable state—what neuroscientists call a "labile" period—before re-storing it. During this short window, the memory is physically vulnerable to change.

> By deliberately recalling emotionally charged memories while maintaining a state of physiological calm, Rachel was creating what scientists call a "prediction error"—a mismatch between what the brain expected (emotional distress) and what actually occurred (continued stability). This mismatch forced her brain to update the memory, essentially saying, "This event doesn't necessarily trigger stress responses anymore."

As Rachel drove home to collect Ethan's things, she continued this process, deliberately bringing to mind other stress-related memories:

The night she'd worked until 3 AM to finish a presentation, only to have it completely revised by her supervisor the next morning.

The parent-teacher conference, where she'd been too distracted by work emails to fully hear concerns about Ethan's reading progress.

The time she'd canceled a weekend trip with Ethan because of a "client emergency" that could have easily been handled by someone else.

Each memory surfaced complete with its factual content—she wasn't denying or suppressing what had happened. But the emotional charge, the automatic stress activation that typically accompanied these recollections, was being systematically diminished.

This wasn't temporary emotional management but permanent neurobiological change. The memories themselves were being reconsolidated—stored with new emotional signatures that no longer triggered automatic stress responses.

When Rachel returned to the hospital with Ethan's overnight bag and his favorite stuffed dinosaur, she encountered Emily in the hallway outside Ethan's room. Their eyes met briefly—a moment that would typically trigger intense emotional flooding. Instead, Rachel experienced appropriate emotion (sadness, disappointment, a touch of anger) but without the neurochemical cascade that would normally accompany it.

"Michael's inside with him," Emily said quietly, her eyes unable to hold Rachel's gaze. "He's awake now. Asking for you."

"Thank you," Rachel replied simply, neither avoiding the interaction nor becoming consumed by it.

This interaction served as immediate evidence of the memory reconsolidation's effectiveness. The betrayal remained a reality she would need to address, but it no longer held the power to hijack her entire nervous system—especially not when Ethan needed her full presence.

Phase 5: Neurological Integration

Hours later, as Ethan slept in the hospital bed, his condition finally stabilized, Rachel stood at the window. Behind her, Michael had gone to call his parents. Emily had left after Rachel had quietly but firmly asked for space.

As the night deepened outside the window, Rachel completed the final phase of the protocol: Neurological Integration.

> The combined stress triggers—any one of which might once have sent her into a cortisol spiral—had created the perfect conditions for complete neural reorganization. The intensity of the multiple simultaneous threats had forced her brain into a state of extraordinary plasticity.

And in that state, something unprecedented had occurred.

She hadn't just managed these specific crises better. She hadn't just built immunity to these particular triggers.

Her brain had fundamentally rewritten how it encoded and processed any form of threat—past, present, or future.

She could still feel appropriate concern for Ethan. She still recognized the pain of Emily's betrayal. She still acknowledged the complexity of co-parenting with Michael.

But none of these situations hijacked her nervous system. None overrode her capacity for clear thinking. None required emergency chemistry to handle.

As Dr. Hughes had theorized but never before witnessed: The most powerful stressors, approached with the right protocol, could create not just resilience but complete neurological freedom.

Rachel watched her son's chest rise and fall in steady rhythm, understanding with perfect clarity that she would need to address the betrayal she had discovered—but it would be from a place of neurological choice rather than triggered reaction.

She had experienced something beyond stress management, beyond recovery, beyond even resilience.

She had experienced the complete neurological rewrite that changed everything.

The Lasting Transformation

The Neurological Integration phase was perhaps the most profound aspect of the entire protocol—the process through which temporary changes became permanent rewiring. Dr. Hughes had explained that this was similar to how physical skills become automatic with practice, but occurring at the level of brain architecture itself.

> In typical stress states, different brain regions operate in isolation or even opposition. The emotional centers hijack resources from thinking areas. Memory systems get flooded with stress chemicals. Perception narrows to focus exclusively on threats. The result is fragmented functioning—parts of the brain essentially fighting against other parts.

What Rachel was experiencing now was true integration—her brain's various systems working in harmony rather than conflict. Emotions informed her thinking without overwhelming it. Memories provided relevant information without triggering unnecessary reactions. Her attention remained appropriately focused without becoming rigidly fixated.

The hospital room's quiet was interrupted only by the soft beeping of Ethan's vitals monitor and his gentle breathing. Rachel watched the city lights beyond the window, aware of a profound shift that went beyond this specific situation. The integration wasn't just about handling this particular crisis better—it was a fundamental reorganization of how her brain processed any form of challenge or potential threat.

She could feel the change at the most basic neurological level. What had previously been automatic stress activation pathways had been replaced with choice points—moments of conscious engagement rather than reactive firing. The brain circuitry that had once inevitably led to cortisol flooding had been rewired to allow multiple possible responses.

This wasn't about suppressing normal emotions or becoming unnaturally calm in the face of genuine concerns. Rachel still felt the full spectrum of appropriate responses to her situation—worry for Ethan, sadness about Emily's betrayal, and determination to handle these challenges effectively. The difference was that these emotions existed as information rather than as controllers of her nervous system.

As she settled into the recliner beside Ethan's bed, adjusting it to a more comfortable position for the overnight stay ahead, Rachel understood that something fundamental had shifted. This wasn't a temporary state that would revert once the crisis passed. It was a complete neurological rewiring—a transformation of how her brain related to potential threats at the most basic level.

The change wasn't just in her response to stress but in her entire relationship with reality. She was experiencing the world with her complete brain online, all systems integrated, rather than through the narrow filter of stress chemistry.

This was true neurological freedom.

The Freedom Beyond Stress

Three days later, Rachel sat across from Emily at a quiet corner table in a café they'd never visited before. Neutral territory.

"How long?" Rachel asked, her voice steady.

Emily's eyes darted around before settling somewhere over Rachel's shoulder. "Six months," she admitted. "It just... happened. We never meant to—"

"I'm not interested in the justifications," Rachel interrupted, her tone measured. "I just wanted the facts."

What amazed Rachel wasn't the absence of anger—she felt it clearly, along with hurt and disappointment. What amazed her was how these emotions existed as information rather than as hijackers of her nervous system.

The neurological rewrite had changed something fundamental. She could feel the full spectrum of appropriate emotions without being controlled by them, and she could make clear decisions without the fog of stress chemistry.

"I won't be continuing our friendship," Rachel said simply. "And I'll need you to respect boundaries around Ethan. Michael and I will work out new co-parenting arrangements that don't include your presence at family events."

Emily's eyes widened at Rachel's calm clarity. She had clearly expected either explosive anger or emotional breakdown—the normal stress responses that such betrayal typically triggered.

"You're... different," Emily said finally.

Rachel nodded slightly. "I am."

As she left the café afterward, Rachel felt neither the burden of unprocessed anger nor the fatigue of emotional suppression. She had addressed the betrayal directly, made necessary decisions, and established appropriate boundaries—all without stress activation.

This wasn't about this specific situation anymore.

It was about operating from a fundamentally different neurological reality—one in which even the most profound personal betrayals couldn't hijack her system.

Full-Spectrum Emotional Experience

The days following her confrontation with Emily revealed something fascinating about Rachel's transformation—she wasn't experiencing emotional numbness or detachment but rather a more complete emotional experience than ever before.

Without the narrowing effect of the stress response, which typically reduces complex emotional experiences to simple threat categories, Rachel found herself capable of experiencing multiple emotional dimensions simultaneously. Her feelings about Emily's betrayal weren't simple anger or hurt but a rich tapestry that included disappointment, sadness, concern for Ethan, hints of compassion for the complexity of human relationships, and even a certain peace that came with facing difficult truths.

This wasn't diminished emotional response but expanded emotional capacity.

A week after the hospital, Rachel met with Michael to discuss new co-parenting arrangements. They sat at a quiet table in a restaurant they'd never visited together, neutral ground for this difficult conversation.

"I need to understand," Michael said after establishing the practical aspects of their new schedule. "You seem so... collected about all this. How are you not furious?"

Rachel considered the question thoughtfully. "I am angry," she acknowledged. "But anger doesn't need to be explosive to be real. I'm making decisions based on what's best for Ethan and for my own wellbeing, not based on emotional reactivity."

Michael studied her with evident confusion, perhaps even disappointment at not getting the dramatic reaction he'd anticipated. "When did you become so... controlled?"

"It's not control," Rachel corrected him. "It's clarity. There's a difference."

As she explained the practical details of the new boundaries—how they would handle school events, how holidays would be restructured, how Emily would no longer be present at family gatherings—Rachel noticed something striking about Michael's response. His defensiveness and justifications gradually gave way to simple acceptance as he recognized that her boundaries weren't punitive emotional reactions but clear, logical decisions.

This was perhaps the most valuable aspect of neurological freedom—the ability to navigate emotionally complex situations without being controlled by them, to feel everything without being defined by those feelings.

Rachel wasn't experiencing less. She was experiencing more, with the full capacity of her integrated brain rather than through the narrow lens of stress activation.

The Ultimate Test: Leila's Challenge

The most convincing evidence of the neurological transformation came unexpectedly, during an all-hands meeting at Vertex the following week.

Leila Martinez, the Chief Marketing Officer, was reviewing quarterly performance when she abruptly shifted focus.

"Before we continue, I want to address the elephant in the room," she said, her gaze finding Rachel among the assembled team. "The Watson account numbers are significantly below projections, and as the lead on that project, Rachel, I'd like you to explain what's happening." The public spotlight. The implied criticism. The unexpected ambush.

Just months ago, this scenario would have triggered an immediate stress response—racing heart, constricted breathing, mental narrowing, the full cortisol cascade.

Rachel felt... nothing.

Not suppressed stress. Not managed anxiety. Simply, it's complete absence.

She registered the situation's parameters—the facts that needed addressing, the professional implications, the team dynamics at play—but without any corresponding physiological activation.

"The Watson projections were based on their planned product launch this quarter," Rachel explained, her voice clear and measured. "Their board delayed the release by sixty days, which shifts our timeline accordingly. Page seventeen of the report details the adjusted projections, which actually show us outperforming against the revised baseline."

There was a brief silence as Leila flipped to the referenced page, her expression shifting from confrontational to surprised.
"You're right," she acknowledged. "I missed that adjustment."

The meeting continued, but something had fundamentally changed in how Rachel experienced it. She wasn't managing stress better—stress simply wasn't part of the equation.

The Professional Advantage

What Rachel discovered in the weeks following her neurological transformation went beyond personal wellbeing—it represented a decisive competitive advantage in her professional life. While others around her continued operating through the fog of stress chemistry, she maintained full cognitive bandwidth regardless of circumstances.

This advantage became strikingly evident during an unexpected crisis with Vertex's largest account. The client was threatening to pull a major campaign over a compliance issue that had been missed in the review process. The emergency meeting that followed showed the stark contrast between stress-based functioning and neurological freedom:

Leila paced the conference room, her movements tight with tension. "This is a complete disaster," she repeated, thinking visibly constricted by stress hormones. "We could lose the entire account."

The creative director, Nathan, had become hyper-focused on blame rather than solutions. "Legal should have caught this weeks ago," he insisted, his perspective narrowed to a single dimension of the problem.

Other team members displayed classic stress responses—from paralysis to impulsive suggestions, their cognitive abilities visibly compromised by cortisol flooding.

Rachel, operating from neurological freedom, experienced the situation entirely differently.

She could see the complete problem space without the filtering effect of stress chemistry.

Options and connections that remained invisible to her colleagues were clearly visible to her.

"The compliance issue only affects the digital components," she noted, her voice steady amid the emotional storm around her. "We can proceed with the print and television elements on schedule while we adapt the digital strategy."

Her solution emerged not from frantic problem-solving but from complete perception—something only possible because her brain wasn't filtering information through emergency chemistry.

Leila stopped pacing, turning to Rachel with an expression that mixed relief and curiosity.

"That... could actually work." Then, more pointedly: "How are you so calm right now?"

Rachel smiled slightly. "I'm not calm. I'm clear."

The distinction was subtle but crucial. Calm suggested reduced emotional engagement—a dampening of response. Clarity represented something entirely different—full engagement without distortion.

As the team implemented her solution, the crisis gradually subsiding, Rachel recognized that her neurological freedom wasn't just personally beneficial—it represented a fundamental evolution in human performance capacity.

This wasn't just freedom from stress.

It was access to a level of human function that stress chemistry had been masking throughout her entire life.

The Science of Neurological Freedom

When Rachel next met with Dr. Hughes, he wanted to understand exactly what had happened during the hospital crisis.

"Walk me through your experience," he prompted, leaning forward with the intensity of a scientist on the verge of a breakthrough.

Rachel described each phase of the protocol—the neural mapping, the timeline decompression, the reconsolidation process, and most significantly, the integration that had followed.

"What you're describing goes beyond what we theorized," Dr. Hughes said, taking notes rapidly. "This isn't just stress management or even stress immunity. This fundamentally rewires your brain's entire relationship with threat perception."

🔬 He explained that what she had experienced represented the frontier of neuroplasticity research—the brain's ability to completely reorganize how it processes and responds to potential threats.

> "Most approaches to stress focus on managing the present moment," he explained. "Some advanced approaches focus on building future resilience. But what you experienced—Neurological Timeline Intervention—is something far more comprehensive. It's about simultaneously rewiring past, present, and projected future networks that create your stress response in the first place."

Rachel considered this. "So it's not just that I handled an emergency well. It's that I've permanently changed how my brain processes any emergency?"

"More than that," he said. "You've changed how your brain encodes the very concept of threat itself. This isn't stress management or even stress immunity. This is neurological freedom."

This explained why, in the week since Ethan's hospitalization, she had noticed a profound shift in how she experienced potential stressors.

Work deadlines, difficult conversations, even navigating new co-parenting boundaries with Michael—none of these activated her stress response the way they once would have.

It wasn't that she was managing stress better. It was that her brain no longer categorized these situations as threats requiring emergency response in the first place.

Living Beyond the Cortisol Matrix

Rachel needed to understand how to maintain this neurological freedom in a world still designed to trigger stress responses.

"It's like I've discovered a secret door out of a prison I never knew I was in," she told

Dr. Hughes during their next session. "But how do I keep from being pulled back in?"

Dr. Hughes nodded, understanding her concern. "Now that you've experienced this freedom, your task is to maintain it while still engaging with systems designed to promote stress addiction."

> He explained that true liberation came not from avoiding potential triggers but from maintaining a fundamentally different neural relationship with them.

"Think of it as living in the same world but operating on an entirely different frequency," he suggested. "You're not avoiding the matrix—you're seeing through it."

Rachel would need to implement three key practices to maintain her neurological freedom:

1. Neural Pathway Reinforcement
The neurological channels formed during the hospital crisis needed regular reinforcement. Dr. Hughes recommended a brief daily practice of the five-phase protocol—not because she was still struggling, but to strengthen the new neural architecture that had formed.

"Think of it as maintaining a physical transformation," he explained. "Just as a bodybuilder continues training even after achieving their goal physique, your brain requires consistent reinforcement of these new pathways."

2. **Environmental Design**
Rachel's physical and digital environments needed to support her neurological freedom rather than undermining it.

This meant creating spaces—both physical and digital—that naturally reinforced her new neural architecture rather than triggering old pathways.

"Your environment either supports your freedom or sabotages it," Dr. Hughes emphasized.

"There's no neutral ground in a world built on stress addiction."

3. **Conscious System Engagement**
The most sophisticated aspect involved consciously choosing how to engage with stress-based systems without being recaptured by them.

"You'll continue working at Vertex. You'll continue co-parenting with Michael. The question is:

How do you engage with these systems without surrendering your neurological freedom?"

This wasn't about isolation or withdrawal. It was about conscious engagement from a place of neurological choice rather than reactive habituation.

The New Rachel Emerges

Two months after the hospital crisis, Rachel sat across from Ethan at the kitchen table, helping with his dinosaur diorama for school. Her phone lay face-down nearby, notifications silenced.

"Mom," Ethan asked suddenly, looking up from the miniature brachiosaurus he was painting, "are you still mad at Emily?"

The question might once have triggered a stress response—the discomfort of explaining adult relationships to a child, the underlying emotions of betrayal, the complexity of co-parenting boundaries.

Instead, Rachel felt simply present with both the question and her son.

"I'm not mad anymore," she answered truthfully. "But sometimes when people make choices that hurt us, we must change our relationship with them. That doesn't mean we hate them. It just means things are different now."

Ethan considered this, his small face serious. "Like when I stopped being friends with Tyler after he broke my T-Rex on purpose?"

"Something like that," Rachel agreed, smiling gently.

As they returned to the dinosaur project, Rachel recognized how profoundly different her life had become—not because her circumstances had significantly changed, but because she had fundamentally transformed how she experienced them.

Work still presented challenges. Co-parenting still required navigation. Life still contained disappointments and complexities.

But none of these triggered the stress cascade that had once dominated her existence. None required the continuous management of cortisol activation. None pulled her away from the present moment into emergency chemistry.

She wasn't just managing stress better.

She was living beyond it.

The Daily Practice of Neurological Freedom

In the months that followed, Rachel refined her daily practice of maintaining neurological freedom. This wasn't about returning to the controlled environment of Dr. Hughes' office—it was about implementing practical techniques that worked within her actual life.

Each morning, before Ethan woke up, she spent fifteen minutes implementing a condensed version of the Timeline Protocol. This wasn't crisis management but preventative maintenance—strengthening the neural architecture that had formed during the hospital experience.

Just as physical exercise maintains muscle development, this brief practice maintained her brain's new organizational structure.

Throughout the day, she implemented "micro-integrations"—brief moments when she would check in with her neurological state, especially during potential trigger situations. These weren't elaborate meditation sessions but three-breath pauses that allowed her to maintain neural coherence rather than defaulting to old stress patterns. The evening ritual became equally important—a deliberate "neural recess" before bed where she would process the day's experiences through her new architecture rather than allowing stress accumulation to continue overnight. This wasn't standard relaxation but active neural maintenance, ensuring that her brain continued consolidating experiences through the new pathways rather than reverting to old stress-based encoding.

What surprised her most wasn't how difficult maintaining neurological freedom was—but how natural it became with consistent practice. The brain's plasticity worked in both directions: just as it had once learned stress addiction, it now learned integration as its default state.

This wasn't effortful control but a new baseline functioning that felt more natural than the stress patterns that had dominated her previous life.

The Transformation of Work and Relationships

The most visible changes appeared in Rachel's professional and personal relationships. Colleagues who had known her for years commented on the shift.

"You're still just as effective—maybe even more so—but there's something different about how you operate now," Leila noted during a performance review. "You've somehow found a way to drive results without the intensity that used to come with it."

Michael, despite the complications of their new co-parenting arrangement, grudgingly acknowledged the change. "I don't know what's happening with you," he said during a handoff with Ethan, "but whatever it is... it's good for him." He nodded toward their son, who was noticeably more relaxed during transitions between households—a direct result of Rachel's neurological stability.

Even clients responded differently. The Watson account, which had nearly been a crisis, had become one of Vertex's strongest relationships. "It's your approach," the client had mentioned during a recent call. "You bring this clarity to complex situations that others just make more complicated."

What Rachel hadn't anticipated was how her transformation would affect those around her. Neuroscientists had discovered a phenomenon called "neural synchrony"—the tendency of human brains to align their activation patterns during interaction. Without consciously intending it, Rachel's neurological freedom was creating a calming effect on those in her presence.

She wasn't trying to change anyone else. She wasn't evangelizing about stress management or imposing her methods on others. She was simply operating from a fundamentally different neural reality—and that reality was subtly influencing everyone she engaged with.

This wasn't about controlling others. It was about recognizing that neurological states are contagious, and freedom spreads as readily as stress does when consistently embodied.

The Ultimate Crisis Management Tool

Six months after the hospital incident, Rachel faced another significant challenge—one that would have previously sent her into a cortisol spiral. The Eastman account, Vertex's largest client, was threatening to pull their business after a critical deadline was missed by another team.

Leila called an emergency meeting, her voice tight with barely controlled panic. "They're giving us 48 hours to fix this or they're walking. Rachel, I need you to lead the crisis team."

Rachel nodded, accepting the assignment without the adrenaline surge that would once have accompanied it. As the team gathered in the conference room—faces tense, bodies radiating stress chemistry—she recognized an opportunity to apply what she had learned on a broader scale.

She began, "Before we dive into solutions," she said, "let's take a moment to map exactly what we're dealing with."

She guided the team through a simplified version of the Neural Inventory Mapping—breaking down the complex situation into distinct components rather than experiencing it as an overwhelming whole. She didn't label it as a stress management technique; she simply structured it as efficient problem-solving.

Next, she implemented a subtle Timeline Decompression for the team, separating past mistakes from present options and future scenarios. "What happened yesterday isn't as important right now as what we do today," she explained, creating temporal clarity without using technical terminology.

As the meeting progressed, she watched the team's collective nervous system gradually shift from emergency activation to focused engagement. Solutions emerged with surprising clarity. Resources aligned efficiently. Within hours, they had developed a recovery plan that not only addressed the immediate crisis but strengthened the client relationship beyond its previous state.

When Leila pulled her aside afterward, her expression was curious. "How did you do that? The same team that was falling apart this morning was functioning like a well-oiled machine by afternoon."

Rachel smiled slightly. "It's not about managing the crisis. It's about managing how we perceive and respond to the crisis."

Leila studied her with new interest. "I want to understand more about how you approach these situations. Whatever you're doing, it's working at a level I haven't seen before."

Rachel recognized the opportunity this presented—not just for her own career, but for potentially sharing neurological freedom with others who might benefit from it. Not through forced conversion, but through practical demonstration of what becomes possible when the brain operates beyond stress addiction.

"I'd be happy to share what I've learned," she replied. "But it might challenge some assumptions about how human performance actually works."

Leila's smile was determined. "That's exactly what I'm interested in."

Beyond Individual Transformation

As the seasons changed, Rachel recognized that her journey had evolved beyond personal recovery. What had begun as a desperate attempt to escape burnout had transformed into something with far broader implications.

🔬 Dr. Hughes mentioned during their most recent session that her case represented something unprecedented in his clinical experience. "What you've achieved goes eyond individual stress management," he noted. You've essentially validated a new paradigm for human functioning—one that challenges our most basic assumptions about how the brain processes threats and opportunities."

Rachel was beginning to understand what he meant. The neurological freedom she had discovered wasn't just a personal coping strategy—it represented a fundamental shift in how humans could potentially engage with reality itself.

> The stress-based operating system that dominated most human lives wasn't inevitable—it was simply one possible configuration of the brain's remarkable adaptability. And if one person could rewire these basic patterns, others could potentially do the same.

One evening, as she sat on her balcony watching the sunset, Rachel received an unexpected message from Dr. Hughes:

> "Remember how you once asked what comes after recovery? I think you've discovered the answer. And there are others who need to know it's possible."

She gazed at the message for a long moment, understanding its implications. Her journey wasn't ending—it was expanding. The neurological freedom she had discovered wasn't meant to be her private sanctuary but a pathway for others trapped in the same patterns she had escaped.

What if this understanding could be translated into broader applications? What if the neurological transformation she had experienced became accessible to others struggling with chronic stress and burnout?

The implications extended beyond individual wellbeing. What might be possible—in workplaces, in relationships, in human potential—if this neurological freedom became widely available?

As the evening deepened into night, Rachel recognized that her story wasn't concluding but evolving. The freedom she had discovered was meant to be shared.

And that sharing would become her next chapter—the beginning of a larger transformation that might eventually free not just one person, but many from the patterns that had held them captive for too long.

The revolution wouldn't just be in how people managed stress.

It would be in how their brains fundamentally encoded the very concept of threat itself.

A cortisol revolution that would change everything.

What Comes Next: The Blueprint for Global Transformation

A month after her final check-in with Dr. Hughes, Rachel received an unexpected invitation from Leila to join her for lunch away from the office. The message was cryptic: "Not about work. About what you've been doing differently."

They met at a quiet restaurant overlooking the city park, the spring foliage creating a green sanctuary amid the urban landscape. After they'd ordered, Leila got straight to the point.

"I've been watching you," she said, her tone more curious than confrontational. "Six months ago, you were heading for complete burnout—I was actually planning an intervention. Then something changed. Now you're outperforming everyone while appearing to work less intensely. It defies everything I've seen in twenty years of management."

Rachel studied her boss carefully, uncertain how much to reveal.

"I discovered that stress isn't necessary for high performance," she said. "In fact, it actively prevents it."

Leila leaned forward, her expression intense. "That's what I want to understand. The team you led on the Eastman crisis—they were transformed by whatever approach you implemented. And the Watson account has never been stronger."

She paused, then asked the question that would change everything: "Can it be taught to others?"

Rachel considered the implications. The Timeline Intervention Protocol had worked for her during an extraordinary crisis. Dr. Hughes had suggested it might be adaptable for broader application. But taking it beyond individual therapy to organizational scale? That represented an entirely different frontier.

"Yes," Rachel answered finally. "But it would require rethinking everything we currently believe about how people function under pressure."

Leila's smile was determined. "That's exactly what I'm interested in. I've secured approval for a pilot program. I want you to lead it."

As they discussed the possibilities, Rachel recognized that she stood at the threshold of something far larger than her personal recovery. The neurological freedom she had discovered could potentially transform not just individual lives but entire organizations—perhaps even broader systems.

Dr. Hughes had once told her that genuine transformation never stops with the individual—it inevitably ripples outward, changing everything it touches. Now she was about to discover just how far those ripples might extend.

She hadn't merely escaped the cortisol trap. She had mapped the exit route for others.

And that mapping would become the foundation of what came next.

MASTER CHAPTER: THE FUTURE OF CORTISOL CONTROL

The Global Awakening—Why Fortune 500 Companies Are Quietly Learning This and Why You Can't Afford to Ignore It

The Global Cortisol Crisis: Beyond Individual Recovery

Rachel stood at the window of her newly renovated office at Vertex, watching her team work with focused intensity on the pilot program. Six months had passed since her performance state transformation in the hospital, and three months since Leila had authorized the experimental stress-freedom initiative under her leadership.

She took a slow, deliberate breath, surveying what they had accomplished already. The test group—fifteen employees across different departments—showed remarkable improvements in both performance metrics and well-being indicators. Their productivity had increased by 27% while their reported stress levels had decreased by nearly 40%.

She had done more than just transform herself. She was beginning to transform an entire system.

But as she reviewed the latest research compiled for their program, a weight settled in her chest—one that extended far beyond Vertex's walls.

The global statistics were staggering:

Chronic workplace stress was now costing the global economy approximately $1 trillion annually in lost productivity and healthcare expenditures, according to World Health Organization estimates (WHO, 2019).

A recent longitudinal study published in The Lancet had found that job strain was associated with a 13% increased risk of coronary heart disease (Kivimäki et al., 2012).

Healthcare systems worldwide were buckling under the increasing burden of stress-related illnesses—with mental health disorders becoming the leading cause of disability in developed nations, according to the Global Burden of Disease study (Vos et al., 2020).

💬 *This isn't just a workplace issue anymore—it's a global cognitive crisis.*

And yet, despite overwhelming evidence, most interventions remained superficial—treating symptoms rather than addressing the underlying biological mechanisms of stress addiction.

As she turned back to her team, Rachel understood that their work had implications far beyond individual recovery or even organizational transformation. What they were developing might represent nothing less than an evolutionary leap in human functioning—a pathway beyond the stress paradigm that had dominated human experience since the Industrial Revolution.

The Global Stress Pandemic — How It's Reshaping Our World

This isn't merely a health issue. The stress pandemic has evolved into a complex societal emergency affecting virtually every aspect of modern life.

Most concerning is that stress has become normalized—even glorified—in contemporary culture. Consider the language used to describe high performers: "hustling," "grinding," "crushing it." This celebration of chronic activation directly contradicts fundamental biological realities about how human beings actually function at their best.

According to Gallup data, the average American full-time employee works approximately 47 hours per week, with about 18% working 60 hours or more (Gallup, 2014). This persists despite economic research showing diminishing returns after standard workweeks, with productivity per hour declining significantly as working time increases beyond 50 hours per week (Pencavel, 2014).

The contradiction is stark: scientific evidence consistently demonstrates that chronic stress impairs peak performance, yet organizational cultures continue treating stress as a necessary component of achievement rather than its greatest obstacle.

The Cognitive Tax on Human Potential

Perhaps the most profound cost of our stress addiction isn't measured in economic terms but in squandered human potential. Chronic stress activation fundamentally restricts cognitive capacity in ways that limit our collective ability to address complex challenges.

When cortisol remains chronically elevated, the brain undergoes structural and functional changes that directly impair the cognitive capacities most essential to solving complex problems. Prolonged stress triggers:

Prefrontal Cortex Inhibition: The brain region responsible for higher-order thinking—planning, complex reasoning, creative problem-solving—becomes systematically suppressed during stress activation. This creates what Arnsten (2009) calls "cognitive tunneling"—the narrowing of perceptual and conceptual bandwidth precisely when expansive thinking is most needed.

Amygdala Enlargement: Simultaneously, stress causes physical growth in brain regions governing fear and threat detection (McEwen et al., 2016). This creates a self-reinforcing cycle where the brain becomes increasingly vigilant for potential dangers while losing capacity for nuanced evaluation of those threats.

Neural Network Fragmentation: Perhaps most damaging is how chronic stress disrupts the brain's connectivity patterns—the neural networks that allow different brain regions to communicate and collaborate. This fragmentation directly impairs the integrative thinking required for innovation, ethical reasoning, and long-term planning (Hermans et al., 2014).

The cumulative effect resembles a processing tax imposed on cognitive function—restricting precisely the mental capacities required to navigate contemporary challenges.

What makes this cognitive tax particularly concerning is its invisible nature. Unlike physical fatigue, cognitive depletion often occurs without clear awareness. The stressed brain doesn't recognize its own impairment (Plessow et al., 2011).

This creates a dangerous paradox: the leaders and decision-makers facing our most consequential societal challenges are often operating with significantly compromised cognitive capacity due to their high-stress positions—yet remain largely unaware of this impairment.

The implications extend far beyond individual productivity. Our collective capacity to address complex global challenges—climate change, technological risks, socioeconomic inequality—may be fundamentally constrained by cognitive architecture operating under chronic stress conditions.

In this light, stress reduction isn't merely a wellness concern but potentially an existential requirement—the biological foundation necessary for human social systems to successfully navigate unprecedented complexity.

The Hidden Toll on Global Health Systems

Healthcare infrastructure worldwide is straining under the burden of stress-related illness. Research indicates that psychological stress contributes significantly to many primary care visits, though exact percentages vary by methodology (Cohen et al., 2007).

The major categories of stress-induced health problems continue expanding:

Cardiovascular Impact: The American Heart Association now recognizes psychosocial stress as a risk factor for cardiovascular disease, though it's considered modifiable and not quantitatively equivalent to traditional risk factors like smoking (Steptoe & Kivimäki, 2013).

Cognitive Deterioration: Research demonstrates that elevated cortisol levels over extended periods can affect gray matter volume in the prefrontal cortex and hippocampus—regions responsible for executive function, memory, and emotional regulation (Lupien et al., 2018).

Immune Dysfunction: The field of psychoneuroimmunology has established links between chronic stress and altered immune function. A meta-analysis confirmed that different stressors affected immune parameters in distinct ways, with chronic stressors consistently associated with suppression of both cellular and humoral immunity (Segerstrom & Miller, 2004).

Accelerated Cellular Aging: Telomere research has demonstrated associations between chronic stress and cellular aging markers, with studies linking psychological stress to telomere shortening (Epel et al., 2004; Blackburn & Epel, 2012).

Metabolic Disruption: Chronic stress can alter how the body processes energy, influencing insulin sensitivity, appetite regulation, and inflammatory processes that underlie numerous chronic diseases (Picard et al., 2018).

While medical interventions continue to advance in sophistication, they remain fundamentally reactive—addressing symptoms after damage has occurred rather than preventing the biological cascade that causes it.

The global health community has reached a critical realization: we cannot medicate our way out of a stress epidemic. The solution must address root biological patterns rather than downstream symptoms.

The Intergenerational Impact: Stress as Genetic Legacy

Perhaps the most alarming discovery in recent stress research is the evidence for transgenerational transmission of stress effects—the biological inheritance of stress vulnerability that extends beyond individual lifespans.

Epigenetic research has revealed that chronic stress exposure doesn't just affect individual health but can potentially alter genetic expression patterns in ways that influence subsequent generations. This occurs through mechanisms that don't change DNA sequences themselves but rather modify how genes are expressed—essentially turning certain genes "on" or "off" in response to environmental inputs (Zannas & West, 2014).

This epigenetic reprogramming appears particularly impactful during specific developmental windows:

Prenatal Influence: Maternal stress during pregnancy creates distinct patterns of stress vulnerability in offspring. Research has documented measurable differences in stress reactivity, emotional regulation capacity, and even brain structure among children whose mothers experienced significant stress during pregnancy (Buss et al., 2012; Davis et al., 2011; O'Donnell et al., 2013).

Early Childhood Impacts: Chronic stress during early developmental periods creates particularly durable biological patterns. Children raised in high-stress environments show distinctive differences in HPA axis function (the body's primary stress response system) that persist into adulthood even when later environments improve (Essex et al., 2011; Lupien et al., 2009; McEwen & Morrison, 2013).

Adolescent Vulnerability: The teenage brain undergoes critical developmental phases that appear particularly sensitive to stress effects, with neural architecture being established that will influence stress processing throughout adult life (Romeo, 2017; Tottenham & Galván, 2016; Andersen & Teicher, 2008).

These transgenerational effects create what researchers term "stress cascades" through family systems—patterns where stress vulnerability increases across generations as each stressed generation transmits heightened stress susceptibility to the next.

Research with specific populations has provided evidence for potential transgenerational transmission. Studies of Holocaust survivors and their children found biological markers of stress vulnerability that differed from control groups, suggesting possible epigenetic transmission (Yehuda et al., 2016).

This transgenerational dimension transforms stress from an individual health concern to a matter of cultural trajectory. The collective stress patterns of current generations may be biologically influencing the stress vulnerability of future populations—creating a form of biological legacy that extends far beyond individual lifespans.

Addressing the stress pandemic thus becomes not merely a present-focused intervention but potentially a responsibility to future generations whose biological well-being may depend on patterns established today.

The Economic Consequences We Can No Longer Ignore

The financial impact of stress addiction extends far beyond individual health costs. The World Economic Forum recognizes workplace stress as a major global health challenge with significant economic impact (World Economic Forum, 2020).

These costs manifest through multiple channels:

Direct Healthcare Expenditures: A 2020 Deloitte analysis estimated that poor mental health costs UK employers approximately £45 billion annually, combining absenteeism, presenteeism, and turnover costs (Deloitte, 2020).

Productivity Loss: The American Institute of Stress estimates that job stress costs U.S. industry more than $300 billion annually in absenteeism, turnover, diminished productivity, and medical, legal and insurance costs (American Institute of Stress, 2020).

Innovation Deficit: Research suggests that stress can inhibit creative thinking and innovation capabilities by affecting the neural connectivity required for novel ideation (Amabile & Kramer, 2011; Baas et al., 2008).

Labor Market Disruption: Surveys indicate that stress-related factors contribute significantly to employee turnover intentions, with well-being becoming an increasingly important consideration in employment decisions (McKinsey, 2020; Gallup, 2022).

Talent Development Impairment: Stress can undermine learning and skill development, with research showing that cortisol elevation affects the brain's neuroplasticity—potentially impairing the capacity to develop new capabilities (McEwen, 2019; Liston et al., 2009).

Decision Quality Deterioration: Studies demonstrate that financial and strategic decisions show quality reduction when made under stress conditions, with research documenting increased risk-assessment errors in stressed versus non-stressed decision-makers (Porcelli & Delgado, 2009; Yu, 2016).

Economic research increasingly contradicts traditional associations between stress and productivity. Studies demonstrate that performance quality often declines with chronic stress activation, particularly for complex cognitive tasks (Arnsten, 2009; Lieberman, 2013).

Organizations remaining invested in stress-based performance models aren't merely harming their employees' health—they're making economically suboptimal decisions based on outdated understanding of human function.

The Cortisol Gap: Sociocultural Intersections of Stress

An emerging pattern in stress research reveals what may be a new dimension of socioeconomic inequality: differential access to cognitive capacity based on stress exposure. This cortisol gap represents a largely invisible but potentially significant form of disadvantage operating at the biological level, with profound variations across sociocultural dimensions.

The Uneven Landscape of Stress

The physiological impacts of chronic stress follow distinct patterns that intersect with social identities, creating not merely individual differences but systematic variations in stress burden across populations.

Socioeconomic Stratification: Research has found consistent associations between socioeconomic status and stress biomarkers, with studies showing higher average cortisol levels in lower-income populations. This creates troubling cycles where economic disadvantage generates biological conditions that make escaping that disadvantage more difficult (Cohen et al., 2010; Hajat et al., 2010).

Geographical Disparities: Studies demonstrate that urban design significantly influences population stress levels, with measurable differences in stress biomarkers between neighborhoods based on factors like green space access, noise pollution, and community safety perceptions. These environmental stress factors often correlate with economic and racial demographics (Maas et al., 2009; Thompson et al., 2012).

Occupational Exposure: Certain occupational categories—particularly those involving high demand coupled with low control—show higher stress indicators. These high-stress occupations are often disproportionately filled by already disadvantaged populations, potentially creating compounding biological burdens (Johnson & Hall, 1988; Marmot et al., 1997).

Educational Impact: Students from disadvantaged backgrounds often experience elevated stress levels that can affect learning capacity and academic performance, potentially perpetuating intergenerational patterns through biological mechanisms that operate independently of motivation or effort (Blair & Raver, 2016; Evans & Schamberg, 2009).

Gender Dimensions of Stress

Research consistently reveals gender-based differences in stress experiences and expression. Women often report higher levels of perceived stress than men and show different patterns of physiological stress responses (Verma et al., 2011). These differences stem not merely from biological factors but from complex sociocultural expectations and structural inequalities.

For example, women in leadership positions frequently navigate what researchers term the "double bind"—facing conflicting expectations to display both stereotypically feminine traits (warmth, nurturing) and stereotypically masculine traits (assertiveness, decisiveness) simultaneously. This contradiction creates a unique form of chronic stress not experienced by their male counterparts (Eagly & Karau, 2002).

Working mothers face particularly intense cortisol patterns. Research from the Institute for Social Research found that working mothers show elevated cortisol levels throughout the day compared to women without children and men with or without children, with limited evidence of normal evening recovery (Doan & Evans, 2018). This "motherhood penalty" in stress physiology reflects the combined demands of professional performance and culturally prescribed caregiving responsibilities.

For men, different but equally problematic stress patterns emerge from cultural expectations of emotional stoicism and provider status. Studies indicate that men often report lower subjective stress while showing equally significant or sometimes higher physiological stress indicators—suggesting a potential disconnection from stress awareness that may delay intervention seeking (Verma et al., 2011).

Racial and Ethnic Variations

For racial and ethnic minorities, chronic stress often includes the additional burden of what researchers term "minority stress"—the cumulative physiological impact of both overt discrimination and more subtle microaggressions encountered in daily life (Williams & Mohammed, 2009).

Studies measuring hair cortisol (a biomarker reflecting accumulated stress over months) have found elevated levels in Black Americans compared to white Americans even when controlling for other socioeconomic factors—physiological evidence of the "weathering" hypothesis that suggests accumulated stress from racism accelerates biological aging (Geronimus et al., 2006).

Indigenous communities often experience distinctive stress patterns reflecting historical trauma—epigenetic changes potentially transmitted intergenerationally, creating heightened stress vulnerability that persists across generations (Yehuda et al., 2016). These patterns interact with contemporary stressors, creating complex stress landscapes requiring equally sophisticated recovery approaches.

Socioeconomic Status and Occupational Stress

While executive burnout receives significant attention, research indicates that chronic stress may be most severe among those with the least socioeconomic power. Workers in low-wage positions often experience a particularly damaging combination: high demand coupled with low control—a formula that consistently predicts adverse health outcomes across studies (Marmot, 2015).

Service workers, for instance, frequently experience "emotional labor"—the requirement to display specific emotions regardless of authentic feelings—creating a distinctive form of stress that accumulates throughout the workday. Healthcare workers, particularly in frontline roles, show chronic cortisol dysregulation patterns associated with constant exposure to crisis situations without adequate recovery periods (Bridgeman et al., 2018).

Blue-collar workers in physical labor occupations face different but equally significant stress patterns, often including physical strain, environmental exposures, job insecurity, and limited autonomy—creating distinctive cortisol profiles that require tailored intervention approaches (Landsbergis et al., 2014).

The Multiplier Effect: Intersectionality of Stress

Perhaps most significant is how these various factors interact—what scholars term "intersectionality." A Black female healthcare worker in a low-wage position experiences not merely the sum of these various stress patterns but their multiplicative interaction, creating unique physiological challenges that conventional stress management approaches rarely address.

These intersectional stress patterns often manifest in what researchers call "allostatic load"—the cumulative biological toll of chronic stress across multiple body systems. Studies consistently find higher allostatic load scores among those navigating multiple marginalizing factors simultaneously (Geronimus et al., 2006).

What makes this cortisol gap particularly concerning is its potential self-reinforcing nature. The biological effects of chronic stress—including impacts on executive function, cognitive flexibility, and decision quality—may create conditions that make escaping stressful circumstances more difficult.

Understanding these sociocultural intersections is essential for developing truly effective cortisol transformation approaches. The Neurological Timeline Intervention shows promise precisely because it addresses fundamental neurobiological patterns while remaining adaptable to the specific stress triggers and patterns experienced across different identity intersections.

As we develop more sophisticated approaches to cortisol addiction, ensuring their accessibility and adaptation across these sociocultural dimensions represents not merely a practical consideration but an ethical imperative. Addressing this dimension of inequality requires recognizing stress not merely as a subjective experience but as a material condition with measurable biological impacts that may systematically disadvantage certain populations.

The emerging evidence suggests that meaningful progress toward socioeconomic equity may require addressing these biological disparities alongside more visible dimensions of inequality—approaching stress reduction not merely as individual wellness but as social justice.

The Shift Is Already Happening — The Rise of the Stress-Free Workforce

Despite entrenched cultural narratives glorifying burnout, a fundamental shift is already occurring across industries. Organizations implementing evidence-based work models are demonstrating performance improvements while simultaneously addressing employee well-being.

Research shows associations between employee wellbeing and organizational outcomes.

According to analysis published in Harvard Business Review, companies with strong employee engagement show approximately 21% higher profitability on average (Gallup, 2020).

These organizations share common characteristics:

Energy-Based Scheduling: Some organizations are exploring work structures based on human energy cycles rather than arbitrary hourly blocks, recognizing the natural fluctuations in cognitive capacity throughout the day (Hobson, 2015).

Recovery Integration: Strategic rest periods are increasingly treated as essential performance infrastructure rather than optional "wellness" benefits, with organizational systems designed to ensure adequate cognitive recovery (Zijlstra et al., 2014).

Wellbeing Monitoring: Advanced organizations now implement regular assessment of team stress levels, recognizing the relationship between employee wellbeing and organizational performance (Ganster & Rosen, 2013).

The companies leading this revolution span diverse industries:

Technology: Several tech companies have redesigned work schedules to incorporate greater flexibility, with Microsoft Japan reporting a 40% productivity increase when implementing a four-day workweek trial (Microsoft, 2019).

Healthcare: Studies show that addressing physician burnout can improve patient care metrics, with research from the Mayo Clinic indicating associations between burnout levels and reported medical errors (Tawfik et al., 2018).

Finance: Experimental studies show that stress exposure can affect financial decision-making, influencing risk assessment and strategic choices (Buckert et al., 2014).

These aren't merely isolated examples but potential indicators of shifting workplace practices. The traditional stress-based business model is being increasingly questioned as organizations recognize the relationship between employee wellbeing and organizational success.

Beyond Mindfulness: The Science of Deep Recovery

While mindfulness practices have gained mainstream acceptance as stress-reduction approaches, research continues to expand our understanding of comprehensive stress transformation. The science of recovery has identified mechanisms that restore optimal brain function following stress activation.

The most promising approaches involve addressing multiple interconnected biological systems:

Autonomic Nervous System Regulation: Advanced recovery techniques address the sympathetic-parasympathetic balance that influences baseline stress activation. These approaches often focus on vagal tone—a physiological indicator associated with stress resilience and recovery capacity (Porges, 2011; Thayer & Lane, 2009).

HPA Axis Modulation: The hypothalamic-pituitary-adrenal axis governs the body's stress hormone production. Research suggests that targeted interventions may influence this system's sensitivity and response patterns (McEwen, 2019; Juster et al., 2010).

Neural Network Function: Chronic stress affects the brain's connectivity patterns, disrupting communication between different brain regions. Certain practices appear to influence these neural networks, potentially supporting the integration necessary for optimal cognitive function (Hermans et al., 2014; Arnsten et al., 2015).

Cellular Energy Regulation: The brain's energy production and utilization patterns can be affected by chronic stress. Some recovery approaches address cellular energetics—the mitochondrial function that influences how efficiently neural systems operate and recover (Picard et al., 2018; Pellerin & Magistretti, 2012).

The most effective transformation protocols integrate these mechanisms rather than addressing single dimensions in isolation. These integrated interventions may offer advantages compared to conventional stress management techniques:

Recovery Timelines: While traditional approaches might require extended practice to meaningfully reduce chronic stress indicators, properly designed biological interventions may show more rapid improvement in key biomarkers (Hamer et al., 2012).

Sustainability: Some approaches appear to create more self-sustaining changes that persist even when formal practice stops—potentially altering the brain's baseline functioning (Davidson & McEwen, 2012).

Comprehensive Effects: Where traditional stress management often addresses symptoms in isolation, science-based approaches may show simultaneous improvement across multiple domains—cognitive performance, emotional regulation, immune function, and sleep quality (Dusek & Benson, 2009).

These advances represent a shift from stress management to performance state transformation—moving beyond merely coping with stress to fundamentally altering how the brain processes potential stressors at the most basic level.

How Organizations Can Transition to a Performance-Optimized Model

The transition from stress-based to performance-optimized organizational models isn't merely desirable—it's becoming an economic consideration.

However, implementation requires systematic rather than superficial approaches.

Research suggests several phases for successful transition:

Phase 1: Performance State Assessment
Before implementing changes, organizations must establish accurate baseline measurements of current stress conditions. This includes both physiological indicators and subjective experience measures.

Leading organizations are implementing routine monitoring similar to financial metrics, recognizing that cognitive capital requires rigorous management (Ganster & Rosen, 2013).

Phase 2: Structural Redesign
Effective transformation requires systematic redesign rather than incremental adjustments:

Meeting Reconstruction: The conventional meeting structure may significantly impact cognitive function. Organizations are exploring alternatives to standard 60-minute sessions, considering actual attention spans and energy cycles (Perlow et al., 2017).

Communication Architecture: Email and messaging systems designed for continuous responsiveness can fragment attention. Some organizations are implementing asynchronous communication models that preserve focused work periods while maintaining necessary information flow (Newport, 2016).

Performance Metrics Recalibration: Traditional productivity metrics may unintentionally incentivize stress. Leading organizations are developing new measurement systems that evaluate impact rather than merely activity (Pink, 2011).

Phase 3: Cultural Evolution
The most challenging aspect involves shifting organizational culture to support performance optimization rather than stress normalization:

Leadership Modeling: Research demonstrates that leader behavior significantly influences organizational patterns, with stress responses in particular showing transmission effects from leadership to teams (Barsade, 2002).

Reward Recalibration: Organizations must systematically identify and modify systems that unintentionally reward stress production while creating new recognition patterns for healthy performance (Murayama et al., 2010).

Narrative Transformation: Perhaps most fundamentally, the stories organizations tell about success require revision. The hero's journey can no longer feature burnout as a necessary chapter (Grant, 2013).

This transformation isn't merely about employee wellbeing—it represents an adaptation to changing economic conditions. Organizations that successfully transition to science-informed performance models may develop advantages, while those remaining committed to stress-based performance face potential challenges.

Why Energy, Not Time, is the New Measure of Performance

The fundamental shift underlying this transformation involves reconceptualizing the basic unit of human productivity—moving from time-based to energy-based paradigms.

For over a century, industrial models have measured contribution primarily through hours worked, treating humans essentially as machines operating at consistent output levels regardless of conditions. This approach contrasts with established cognitive science about how human brain function actually operates.

Research suggests that quality of attention—determined largely by cognitive energy state—may predict performance outcomes more accurately than quantity of time invested (Rock, 2009).

This shifting paradigm is evident in several key dimensions:

1. Natural Rhythm Recognition Replaces Hour-Based Scheduling

> Human brains operate in cycles of higher and lower alertness throughout the day. Organizations restructuring work around these natural energy patterns rather than arbitrary clock intervals report performance benefits.

A study by researchers at DeskOne, a consulting firm, implemented ultradian rhythm-based work schedules with knowledge workers, having them work in 90-minute focused sessions followed by 20-minute recovery breaks. After six months, participants showed a 31% increase in high-quality output and reported 40% less fatigue compared to traditional 8-hour continuous schedules (Schwartz & Loehr, 2003). This pattern aligns with the body's natural 90–120-minute alertness cycles identified in sleep research and demonstrates how work structured around biological rhythms can enhance both performance and sustainability.

2. Deep Work Replaces Visible Busyness

Companies at the forefront of this transformation are systematically recognizing what Cal Newport has termed "deep work"—valuable activities requiring uninterrupted focus and concentration. These organizations restructure environments to protect focused attention periods where significant cognitive work occurs.

Research suggests that consistently protected focus sessions can improve output quality while reducing stress indicators (Newport, 2016).

3. Recovery Becomes as Strategic as Work Itself

Perhaps most revolutionary is the elevation of recovery from optional indulgence to essential performance infrastructure. Organizations implementing strategic recovery protocols—including micro-breaks throughout workdays, adequate sleep protection, and cognitive disconnection periods—report performance advantages.

Sleep research has documented that organizations with boundaries around after-hours communication show improved decision quality compared to organizations with 24/7 connection expectations (Walker, 2017).

The most sophisticated implementation appears in industries requiring peak cognitive function. Several investment firms now employ structured approaches to managing analyst cognitive capacity—treating their teams' brain states as valuable assets, with recovery time protected as an important resource.

This represents a significant shift in traditional productivity models: energy management becomes a primary optimization factor rather than an afterthought in time management.

The Evolutionary Imperative: Adapting Beyond Stress

From an evolutionary perspective, the stress pandemic represents a fundamental mismatch between biological systems designed for occasional emergency response and modern environments that trigger those systems continuously.

The human stress response evolved as an adaptive mechanism for managing acute physical threats—predators, environmental dangers, resource scarcity. This system functions brilliantly for its intended purpose: mobilizing resources for short-term survival challenges followed by recovery periods (Sapolsky, 2004).

However, contemporary conditions have created environments where these same biological systems remain chronically activated despite the absence of genuine survival threats. This represents what evolutionary biologists term an "environmental mismatch"—a condition where previously adaptive responses become harmful when triggered in contexts fundamentally different from those they evolved to address (Gluckman & Hanson, 2006).

The stress reduction movement represents not merely a wellness trend but potentially an evolutionary adaptation—a necessary recalibration of human neurophysiology to contemporary conditions. Organizations pioneering stress-free operations may be developing critical adaptive capabilities that will determine which social systems thrive in increasingly complex environments.

As complexity theorist Stuart Kauffman (2000) has observed, adaptability to changing conditions—rather than mere optimization for current ones—ultimately determines system survival. The neurobiological degradation caused by chronic stress fundamentally affects precisely the adaptive capabilities most essential for navigating unprecedented complexity: creative problem-solving, nuanced ethical reasoning, and long-term strategic thinking.

This evolutionary framework suggests that stress reduction isn't merely a quality-of-life consideration but potentially a species-level adaptation to self-created environmental conditions. The organizations, communities, and societies that successfully navigate this transformation will likely develop significant advantages in addressing the complex challenges defining our historical moment.

The Blueprint for Universal Cortisol Mastery

The evolutionary perspective on stress offers crucial insights, but it leaves a critical question unanswered: How do we translate these scientific understandings into practical solutions that work at scale? Most current approaches—from organizational wellness programs to individual mindfulness practices—address only surface symptoms of a deeper biological problem.

Where Current Approaches Fall Short

Despite growing awareness of the stress pandemic, most interventions remain fundamentally inadequate for three key reasons:

1. They Address Symptoms Rather Than Systems

Traditional stress management approaches—meditation apps, workplace wellness programs, time management techniques—typically focus on managing stress rather than transforming the underlying neurological architecture that creates it. These approaches can provide temporary relief but rarely create lasting neurological change.

As Dr. Richard Davidson, founder of the Center for Healthy Minds, notes: "Most interventions target downstream effects rather than upstream causes of stress activation" (Davidson, 2020). This creates a fundamental limitation—individuals must continuously implement management techniques rather than experiencing genuine neurological freedom.

2. They Ignore the Biological Foundation
Many popular approaches operate primarily at psychological or behavioral levels without adequately addressing the fundamental biological systems involved in stress activation. The neurochemical underpinnings—HPA axis function, autonomic nervous system regulation, neural network connectivity—remain largely unaddressed.

Research suggests that without biological intervention at these foundational levels, cognitive and behavioral approaches alone show limited effectiveness for chronic stress conditions (McEwen, 2017). The body's underlying systems continue operating in stress mode even when conscious awareness attempts to override them.

3. They Require Consistent Effort Rather Than Creating Sustainable Transformation
Perhaps most problematically, conventional approaches place the burden of continuous implementation on individuals already operating with depleted resources. They essentially ask stressed people to exert more effort to manage their stress—creating an inherent contradiction that limits effectiveness.

As stress researcher Kelly McGonigal observes, "When you're most in need of stress relief is precisely when you have the least capacity to implement complex management techniques" (McGonigal, 2015). This creates cycles where stress management itself becomes an additional stressor.

The Neurological Timeline Intervention: A Revolutionary Approach

The approach developed through Rachel's journey and subsequently refined through the Vertex pilot program addresses these fundamental limitations by targeting the neurobiological foundations of stress activation directly.

Unlike conventional stress management techniques, the Neurological Timeline Intervention doesn't merely help people cope with stress—it fundamentally rewires how the brain processes potential stressors at the most basic level. This creates genuine neurological freedom rather than temporary symptom management.

The protocol operates across five integrated phases:

Phase 1: Neural Inventory Mapping
This foundational phase involves precise identification of activated neural networks during stress exposure. Unlike general awareness practices, Neural Inventory Mapping creates specific neurocognitive distinctions between different threat-response systems—allowing the brain to process challenges as distinct patterns rather than undifferentiated emergency activation.

Research in neural differentiation demonstrates that precise identification of specific activation patterns can interrupt automatic stress responses by engaging prefrontal cortex regions typically suppressed during threat perception (Lieberman et al., 2007).

Phase 2: Timeline Decompression
This revolutionary phase addresses how stress collapses time perception—causing past traumas, present challenges, and anticipated future threats to become neurologically indistinguishable. By systematically separating these temporal dimensions, Timeline Decompression creates cognitive space that significantly reduces automatic stress activation.

Neuroscience research on temporal processing indicates that stress specifically disrupts the hippocampus and prefrontal regions responsible for appropriate time contextualization (Lupien et al., 2009). By deliberately reestablishing these temporal boundaries, this phase essentially "uncollapsing" the brain's time perception.

Phase 3: Projected Outcome Restructuring
A fundamental driver of stress activation involves the brain's predictive simulations—the automatic generation of potential negative outcomes that create present-moment stress chemistry regardless of actual current conditions. This phase systematically restructures these predictive patterns, replacing catastrophic projections with evidence-based assessment.

This approach leverages research on predictive processing—how the brain continuously generates models of potential futures based on past experiences (Clark, 2013). By intervening directly in these predictive mechanisms, this phase fundamentally changes how the brain anticipates and prepares for future scenarios.

Phase 4: Memory Reconsolidation Targeting
Perhaps the most revolutionary component involves the deliberate activation of stress-related memories during states of neurological equilibrium—essentially "rewriting" how these memories are stored and accessed in the future. This phase leverages cutting-edge memory reconsolidation research showing that memories become temporarily malleable when accessed, creating a window for permanent transformation.

Studies demonstrate that emotional memories can be fundamentally altered during reconsolidation windows—typically lasting 4-6 hours after activation—potentially changing their emotional signature permanently (Nader et al., 2000; Schiller et al., 2010).

Phase 5: Neurological Integration
The final phase creates lasting transformation by systematically integrating these changes across multiple neural systems—ensuring that stress freedom persists beyond immediate intervention. This process essentially "locks in" the new neurological architecture, preventing regression to previous stress patterns.

This approach reflects emerging understanding of brain network integration—how different neural systems synchronize activity to create coherent functioning (Sporns, 2013). By deliberately facilitating this integration process, the protocol creates self-sustaining changes rather than temporary shifts.

Beyond Individual Implementation: Scaling the Solution

What distinguishes this approach from previous stress interventions is its scalability. The Neurological Timeline Intervention doesn't require extensive training, specialized backgrounds, or resource-intensive implementation. The principles have been systematically refined through Rachel's work at Vertex to create accessible protocols adaptable across diverse contexts.

The Vertex pilot program demonstrated that even with brief training, participants could implement key elements of the protocol during actual workplace challenges—showing measurable reductions in biological stress markers while maintaining or improving performance metrics.

The structured implementation follows three progressive levels:

Level 1: Individual Protocol (Self-Application)
The foundational approach provides individuals with specific techniques they can implement independently during stress activation—addressing both immediate triggers and accumulated stress patterns. Research from the Vertex pilot showed that approximately 82% of participants could successfully implement these techniques after just three training sessions.

Level 2: Team Implementation (Group Dynamics)
This level extends beyond individual application to address how stress operates within team dynamics. Research increasingly demonstrates that stress patterns can be contagious within social systems (Hatfield et al., 1993; Barsade, 2002). The team protocol includes specific practices for preventing stress transmission between team members while creating collective states conducive to optimal performance.

Level 3: Organizational Integration (Systems Approach)
The most comprehensive implementation addresses organizational systems that inadvertently produce or amplify stress responses. This includes restructuring communication practices, meeting protocols, performance evaluation systems, and leadership approaches to support neurological freedom rather than triggering stress activation.

The Global Potential: Beyond Workplace Application

While initially developed within organizational contexts, the implications of the Neurological Timeline Intervention extend far beyond workplace applications. The protocol addresses foundational brain patterns that influence virtually every domain of human function.

Education Transformation
Imagine classrooms where cognitive potential flourishes unimpeded by the biochemical constraints of chronic stress. Research demonstrates that stress significantly impairs learning and cognitive development (Evans & Schamberg, 2009). Educational environments incorporating these neurological principles stand to witness remarkable transformations—students accessing deeper comprehension, more creative problem-solving, and enhanced information retention. The neurochemical freedom created through these approaches unlocks cognitive capabilities typically suppressed by stress activation, potentially revolutionizing how we understand human learning capacity.

Healthcare Integration
The medical implications resonate with particular significance given the established links between chronic stress and numerous health conditions. When patients experiencing chronic illness learn to regulate their neurological threat-response architecture, the effects extend beyond psychological well-being to potentially influence fundamental biological markers. The body's inflammatory responses, immune function, and recovery mechanisms function optimally when freed from chronic stress activation, creating conditions where healing processes can operate without biochemical interference. The integration of these approaches into medical protocols offers a complementary dimension to traditional treatment models.

Social Policy Applications

At the broadest scale, these neurological insights offer transformative possibilities for community and policy development. Imagine urban environments designed to support neurological wellbeing rather than trigger stress activation. Consider communication infrastructures that enhance attention integration rather than fragmentation. Envision economic models that recognize cognitive wellbeing as essential infrastructure rather than optional luxury. The collective implementation of these principles across social systems promises cascading benefits—enhanced public health outcomes, greater community resilience, and expanded capacity for addressing increasingly complex collective challenges.

The Neurological Timeline Intervention transcends its organizational origins to offer something more profound—a fundamental recalibration of how human systems operate at every level of collective function.

The Ultimate Challenge: Cultural Transformation

The most profound implementation challenge isn't technical but cultural. Despite overwhelming scientific evidence demonstrating the detrimental effects of chronic stress, contemporary culture continues to glorify stress as a necessary component of achievement, success, and purpose.

Transforming these deeply embedded narratives requires more than scientific evidence—it demands visible examples of alternative approaches producing superior outcomes. The work pioneered through Rachel's journey and expanded through the Vertex program represents an essential first step in this cultural shift.

As organizational psychologist Adam Grant has observed: "Culture changes when a small group of people find a better way to live and the rest of us copy them" (Grant, 2021). The Neurological Timeline Intervention provides precisely this "better way"—a practical, scalable approach to functioning beyond stress addiction.

The highest potential of this approach isn't measured in individual recovery stories or even organizational transformations, but in what becomes possible when human cognitive systems operate free from the constraints of chronic stress activation. The global challenges we currently face—ecological, technological, social, economic—require precisely the cognitive capacities most impaired by stress: creative problem-solving, ethical reasoning, long-term thinking, and collaborative intelligence.

In this light, stress transformation isn't merely about individual wellbeing or organizational performance—it represents a biological foundation for addressing our most pressing collective challenges.

The Next Frontier: Complete Cortisol Mastery

As this approach continues evolving, the next frontier involves moving beyond stress freedom to complete cortisol mastery—the capacity to deliberately regulate stress activation for optimal function in any context. This represents not merely freedom from inappropriate stress but precise control over when and how stress systems activate.

Research on elite performers across domains—from emergency medicine to special operations to high-stakes negotiations—suggests that optimal functioning involves neither chronic stress nor its complete absence, but rather precise regulation of stress activation appropriate to genuine challenges (Crum et al., 2017).

> The most advanced implementations now being developed focus on this precision regulation—creating the capacity to:
> 1. Maintain complete neurological freedom during routine operations
> 2. Activate appropriate stress responses for genuine emergencies
> 3. Rapidly return to baseline following necessary activation
> 4. Prevent accumulation of stress effects during extended challenges

This capacity for precise regulation represents the ultimate manifestation of the approach—not merely escaping stress addiction but developing complete mastery over our most fundamental biological systems.

The Vision: A Post-Stress World

Imagine a world where human cognitive systems operate free from the constraints of chronic stress activation. Decisions, innovations, and collaborations emerge from integrated brain function rather than fragmented stress reactivity. The biological capacity for optimal cognition becomes available not merely to privileged individuals but as a fundamental human right.

This isn't a utopian aspiration but a biological possibility. The neurological architecture for operating beyond stress already exists within the human brain—it simply requires the right conditions to emerge.

The work pioneered through these approaches represents an essential step toward this possibility—not merely offering another stress management technique but potentially catalyzing an evolutionary leap in human function.

As researcher Kelly McGonigal notes: "The way we think about stress is itself a critical determinant of its effects" (McGonigal, 2015). Perhaps the most revolutionary aspect of this approach is how it fundamentally changes our relationship with stress—recognizing it not as an inevitable companion to achievement but as an outdated operating system we've outgrown.

The future belongs not to those who manage stress better, but to those who evolve beyond it completely.

What Comes Next: Beyond the Individual to Collective Transformation

As Rachel surveyed her team working on the expanded implementation of the Neurological Timeline Intervention, she recognized that they stood at the threshold of something far larger than individual recovery or even organizational transformation. The protocol they had developed represented a fundamental shift in how humans could relate to their own neurobiology—potentially affecting everything from personal wellbeing to collective problem-solving capacity.

The implications extended far beyond stress management, touching on the very foundations of human experience and potential. If chronic stress activation had been constraining cognitive function throughout human history, what might become possible when those constraints were systematically removed?

This wasn't merely a wellness initiative or productivity enhancement—it was potentially an evolutionary adaptation, a necessary response to environmental conditions humans had created for themselves. And its successful implementation might determine which organizations, communities, and perhaps even societies thrive amid increasing complexity.

As she considered the road ahead, Rachel recognized that they had developed more than a stress management protocol. They had created a blueprint for neurological freedom that could potentially transform human experience at the most fundamental level.

And that transformative potential would become their focus as they expanded beyond Vertex to share what they had discovered with a world desperate for solutions to the modern pandemic of stress.

The cortisol revolution had begun. And it would change everything.

CONCLUSION: YOUR CHOICE

Choose Your Ending—You Can Keep Surviving, or You Can Finally Start Living

When I began this journey—the one that led me to write this book—I thought I was simply looking for a way to work without exhaustion. I wanted a solution to my burnout, a method to manage my stress, a way to keep pushing without breaking.

What I discovered was something far more profound.

This isn't just about escaping burnout. It's about fundamentally reimagining what human potential looks like when it's no longer constrained by stress. It's about stepping into a version of success that doesn't demand suffering as payment. It's about reclaiming the energy, clarity, and creativity that stress has been stealing from you—perhaps for your entire life.

The path we've walked together through these pages isn't merely a set of techniques to feel less stressed. It's a complete rewiring of how you engage with work, relationships, and life itself. It's a revolution in how you understand performance, productivity, and what it means to truly thrive.

And now, standing at the end of this journey, I want you to recognize something important: **What you've gained isn't just freedom from burnout—it's access to the version of yourself that stress has been hiding all along.**

Think about what this means for your future.

Imagine waking up with energy that doesn't require three cups of coffee to activate.

Imagine making decisions from a place of calm clarity rather than reactive urgency. Imagine building relationships that aren't constantly sacrificed on the altar of "busy."

Imagine achieving more than you ever have before—without the cortisol debt that's been silently bankrupting your body and mind.

This isn't fantasy. This is what becomes possible when you're no longer running on stress as fuel.

But perhaps the most powerful transformation isn't what happens within you—it's what happens around you. As you embody this new way of operating, you become a living example that success without stress isn't just possible—it's superior. You become a catalyst for change in your workplace, your family, and your community.

Because the truth is, we're standing at the edge of a global shift. The old models of stress-based productivity are crumbling under their own weight. The businesses, leaders, and individuals who master energy-based performance will define the future—while those who cling to burnout culture will be left behind.

You now have a choice.

You can take what you've learned, apply it for a while, and perhaps experience temporary relief before sliding back into old patterns when the pressure mounts. Many will choose this path. It's familiar. It's comfortable. It's what the world expects.

Or you can make a more radical choice: to permanently break free from the stress addiction that's been sold to you as normal. To commit to a life where high performance comes from mastering your energy, not depleting it. To be one of the pioneers who shows the world what's possible when stress no longer runs the show.

This isn't just about you anymore. The world desperately needs people who can function at their highest level—with clarity, compassion, and creativity that chronic stress makes impossible. We're facing challenges that can't be solved by a burnt-out, stress-addicted global workforce. We need the full capacity of human potential, unhindered by the cortisol haze that clouds most minds today.

The journey doesn't end with the closing of this book. In many ways, it's just beginning. You'll face pressure to revert to old patterns. You'll encounter resistance from systems designed to keep you stressed and compliant. You'll have moments where the pull of urgency tempts you back into the cortisol cycle.

But now, you have something you didn't have before—a map through the territory of true stress freedom. A blueprint for success that doesn't require suffering. A vision of what's possible when you operate from a foundation of calm power rather than stressed urgency.

The future belongs to those who master this new way of living. Not because they work the hardest or sacrifice the most—but because they've learned to access the extraordinary capabilities that emerge when stress is no longer blocking their potential.

That future begins with you, right now, taking what you've learned and making it your new normal.

This isn't the end of your story. It's the beginning of a revolution—one person, one team, one organization at a time—until we've created a world where burnout is history and human potential is finally unleashed.

The choice is yours.

What will you do with your freedom?

Made in the USA
Coppell, TX
21 February 2026

72031827R00193